MASTERING DIFFERENTIAL DIAGNOSIS

A Clinical Approach to Unravelling Complex Cases

BOOK 1

DR KESHAVA BALAJI

notionpress.com

INDIA • SINGAPORE • MALAYSIA

ISBN 979-8-90431-372-2

Contents

Chapter One

Differential Diagnosis of Cardiopulmonary Diseases

Dr. Vijaysekar P.

Differential Diagnosis of Chest Pain

Chest pain is a common and often alarming symptom, prompting millions of visits to emergency departments and primary care physicians each year. Its diverse origins, ranging from benign musculoskeletal issues to life-threatening cardiac emergencies, pose a significant diagnostic challenge. Understanding the pathophysiology of chest pain, recognizing its key presenting features, and systematically approaching the differential diagnosis are crucial for timely and effective management. This article will delve into the complexities of chest pain, exploring its various causes, diagnostic strategies, and critical red flags.

Introduction to Chest Pain: Epidemiology and Significance

Chest pain is a frequent complaint, with a substantial impact on healthcare systems worldwide. It accounts for a significant proportion of emergency department visits, highlighting its prevalence and the associated anxiety it generates. The reasons for this high incidence are multifactorial, encompassing the broad spectrum of potential underlying causes.

Epidemiologically, the prevalence of chest pain varies considerably based on age, sex, and underlying risk factors. For example, cardiac causes are more prevalent in older populations, particularly those with pre-existing conditions like hypertension, diabetes, and hyperlipidemia. Women may present with atypical symptoms of cardiac chest pain, complicating diagnosis. Moreover, the increasing prevalence of conditions such as obesity and sedentary lifestyles has contributed to the rise in both cardiovascular and non-cardiovascular causes of chest pain.

The significance of chest pain lies in its potential to signal severe, life-threatening conditions, particularly acute coronary syndromes (ACS) and pulmonary embolism (PE). Delays in diagnosis and treatment for these entities can result in significant morbidity and mortality. Therefore, a thorough and systematic approach to chest pain evaluation is paramount to identify and manage critical conditions promptly while avoiding unnecessary interventions for benign etiologies.

Pathophysiology of Chest Pain: A Multifaceted Perspective

The sensation of chest pain arises from the stimulation of nociceptors (pain receptors) in various tissues within the thoracic cavity. The diverse origins of chest pain reflect the complexity of these tissues and organ systems, including:

- Cardiac: Pain originating from the heart muscle or its surrounding structures often arises from ischemia (lack of blood supply), inflammation, or mechanical abnormalities. Ischemic pain is typically caused by an imbalance between oxygen supply and demand, triggering nociceptors in the myocardium, or heart muscle. Conditions like ACS, angina, and pericarditis can lead to cardiac chest pain.
- Pulmonary: Chest pain of pulmonary origin is usually associated with irritation or inflammation of the pleura (lining of the lungs), airways, lung parenchyma, or the pulmonary vasculature. Pain can arise from conditions such as pleuritis, pulmonary embolism, pneumonia or pneumothorax. Inflammation or stretching of lung tissue can also trigger nociceptors and cause pain.

- Musculoskeletal: Chest pain stemming from musculoskeletal structures is caused by inflammation, injury, or strain in muscles, bones, joints, or soft tissues of the chest wall. This includes conditions like costochondritis, rib fractures, and muscle strains. These pains are usually triggered by movement or pressure.
- Gastrointestinal: Pain arising from the gastrointestinal tract is often a result of mucosal irritation, esophageal spasms, or inflammation of surrounding organs. Conditions like GERD, peptic ulcers, and esophagitis can cause chest pain through irritation of sensory nerves in the esophagus or upper abdomen.
- Psychological: Psychological factors can contribute to chest pain, particularly in conditions like panic disorder and anxiety. These pains are often thought to be a result of heightened sensitivity to bodily sensations or the physiological effects of panic or anxiety such as muscular tension, rapid heart rate and hyperventilation.

Understanding these different pathophysiological mechanisms is vital for narrowing down the differential diagnosis and guiding the selection of appropriate investigations.

Key Presenting Features of Chest Pain: A Detailed Exploration

A thorough evaluation of chest pain necessitates a detailed history, focusing on key presenting features. These characteristics can provide valuable clues to the underlying cause.

- Onset: The mode of onset can provide insights about the possible underlying cause.
    - Sudden onset: This may suggest conditions like aortic dissection, pulmonary embolism, or pneumothorax.
    - Gradual onset: A gradual onset can be seen in conditions like stable angina, pericarditis, or musculoskeletal pain.

- Location: Describing the site of pain is vital.
    - Central chest pain: Pain in the center of the chest may indicate conditions of cardiac origin like angina or unstable angina.
    - Lateral chest pain: Pain on one side can be suggestive of pulmonary disorders, such as pleuritis or pneumothorax.
    - Specific point tenderness: Localized pain with tenderness may indicate musculoskeletal issues like costochondritis or rib fractures.
- Radiation: Where the pain radiates to gives important clues.
    - Radiation to the arm, jaw, or back: This is often seen with cardiac chest pain, especially ACS.
    - Pleuritic chest pain: Usually does not radiate, but may be well defined in the affected area.
- Character: The quality of the pain provides vital clues.
    - Crushing, squeezing, or tightness: This is usually seen in cardiac chest pain, especially angina or myocardial infarction.
    - Sharp, stabbing, or pleuritic: These are descriptions of pulmonary or pericardial, chest pain that often worsens with breathing.
    - Aching or dull: Musculoskeletal chest pain is often described as dull or aching pain
    - Burning: Burning pain can be indicative of gastrointestinal issues like GERD or esophagitis.
- Intensity: Assessing the pain level using a scale (e.g., 1-10).
    - Severe chest pain is often seen in medical emergencies, such as ACS, aortic dissection, and pulmonary embolism.
    - Mild to moderate chest pain can be seen in many conditions such as musculoskeletal chest pain or anxiety.

- Aggravating/Relieving Factors: Identifying factors that worsen or alleviate the pain is vital.
    - Exertion-induced pain: This is suggestive of angina. Symptoms that disappear with rest are also indicative of angina.
    - Positional changes: Pain worsened by lying down and improved by sitting upright, leans more towards pericarditis. Musculoskeletal pain may worsen with movement.
    - Food related pain: Chest pain that occurs after meals can be due to gastrointestinal causes.
- Associated Symptoms: The presence of other symptoms accompanying chest pain can offer clues to the diagnosis.
    - Shortness of breath: May suggest cardiac, pulmonary, or respiratory problems.
    - Sweating, nausea, vomiting: These are frequently seen in acute coronary syndromes (ACS).
    - Cough, fever, and sputum production: May indicate pulmonary infections like pneumonia.
    - Heartburn or acid reflux: Suggestive of gastroesophageal reflux disease (GERD).
    - Palpitations: Can be associated with cardiac arrhythmias, anxiety, or hyperthyroidism.
    - Dizziness or light-headedness: May indicate a hemodynamic problem or cardiac cause.
    - Anxiety, panic attacks: These may suggest psychogenic chest pain.

A meticulous assessment of these features, along with the patient's medical history, provides essential information for establishing a differential diagnosis.

Differential Diagnosis of Chest Pain: A Detailed Categorization

Chest pain differential diagnosis is broad and encompasses several possible causes. Below, we classify them based on their origin:

Cardiac Chest Pain

- Acute Coronary Syndromes (ACS):
    - ST-Elevation Myocardial Infarction (STEMI): This occurs due to complete occlusion of a coronary artery, leading to myocardial necrosis. STEMI is characterized by ST-segment elevation on ECG accompanied by severe, crushing chest pain, sweating, nausea, and shortness of breath. It is a life-threatening emergency that requires immediate intervention.
    - Non-ST-Elevation Myocardial Infarction (NSTEMI): This also results from myocardial ischemia and necrosis, but usually due to partial coronary artery occlusion. NSTEMI can present with chest pain similar to STEMI, but without ST-segment elevation on ECG. However, it typically shows elevated cardiac enzymes.
    - Unstable Angina: This is a condition where angina symptoms are new in onset, increasing in severity, or occurring at rest. It is a sign of increased risk for myocardial infarction and should be managed aggressively.
    - Pathophysiology: Atherosclerosis, plaque rupture, thrombus formation, myocardial ischemia, cell necrosis, release of cardiac enzymes.

- Stable Angina Pectoris: This is chest pain caused by inadequate blood flow to the heart muscle during physical exertion. Symptoms often resolve with rest or nitro-glycerine. It is typically characterized by predictable chest pain that occurs with exercise or stress and is relieved with rest or medication.

    - Pathophysiology: Imbalance between myocardial oxygen supply and demand and occurs when there is a narrowing of coronary arteries.

- Pericarditis: This is an inflammation of the pericardium, the sac surrounding the heart. It manifests as sharp, pleuritic chest pain that is often worsened by deep breathing, coughing, or lying down, and it is relieved by sitting up and leaning forward.
    - Pathophysiology: Inflammation of the pericardium, potentially caused by viral, bacterial or autoimmune causes.
- Myocarditis: This is an inflammation of the heart muscle, frequently caused by viral infections. It can present with chest pain, shortness of breath, palpitations, and fatigue.
    - Pathophysiology: Inflammation of the myocardium caused by viral infections, autoimmune disorders, or other inflammatory process.
- Aortic Dissection: This is a life-threatening condition involving a tear in the inner lining of the aorta. It presents as severe, tearing chest pain that may radiate to the back.
    - Pathophysiology: A tear in the inner layer of the aorta that can lead to blood flowing into the space between layers.
- Hypertrophic Cardiomyopathy (HCM): A genetic condition characterized by thickening of the heart muscle that can cause chest pain (often exertional), shortness of breath, and arrhythmias.
    - Pathophysiology: An abnormal thickening of the heart muscle, leading to increased stiffness and decreased cardiac output.
- Mitral Valve Prolapse (MVP): This is a common condition where the mitral valve leaflets bulge backward during heart contractions. While often asymptomatic, MVP can cause chest pain, palpitations, and fatigue in some individuals.

    - Pathophysiology: An abnormal displacement of the mitral valve leaflets into the left atrium during heart contraction.

- Prinz metal Angina: This is a variant form of angina caused by coronary artery spasm. It can occur at rest and is often associated with ST-segment elevation on ECG.
    - Pathophysiology: Spasms of the coronary arteries that limit blood flow to the heart.

Pulmonary Chest Pain

- Pulmonary Embolism (PE): This life-threatening condition involves a clot blocking a pulmonary artery, which can cause sudden onset of sharp chest pain, shortness of breath, and haemoptysis (coughing up blood).
    - Pathophysiology: A blood clot that travels into the pulmonary artery, causing obstruction and decreased blood flow to the lungs.
- Pleuritis: This is an inflammation of the pleura, the lining of the lungs. It manifests as sharp, stabbing, pleuritic chest pain that is worsened by breathing, coughing, or movement. Pleuritis can be caused by various conditions including pneumonia, viral infection and autoimmune diseases.
    - Pathophysiology: Inflammation of the pleura, usually caused by infections or inflammatory diseases.
- Pneumothorax: This occurs when air leaks into the space between the lung and chest wall, causing lung collapse. It can result in sudden, sharp chest pain and shortness of breath.
    - Pathophysiology: Air in the pleural space that causes collapse of part of or the entire lung.

- Pulmonary Hypertension: This is a condition involving increased pressure in the pulmonary arteries, leading to right heart strain. It can present with chest pain, shortness of breath, and fatigue.
    - Pathophysiology: An elevation of blood pressure in the pulmonary arteries that lead to increased strain on the right side of the heart.
- Tracheobronchitis: This involves inflammation of the trachea and the bronchi, and can cause substernal chest pain, cough, and sputum production.
    - Pathophysiology: Inflammation of the trachea and bronchi, often caused by a viral infection.
- Lung Cancer: Lung cancer, especially central tumors in the airways, can cause chest pain, coughing and potentially hemoptysis.
    - Pathophysiology: Abnormal cellular growth of lung tissue that leads to tumors.

Gastrointestinal Chest Pain

- Esophageal Spasm: This refers to painful contractions of the muscles in the esophagus. It can cause sudden onset of severe, squeezing chest pain.
    - Pathophysiology: Uncoordinated and intense contractions of the esophageal muscles.
- Gastroesophageal Reflux Disease (GERD): This is a chronic condition characterized by reflux of gastric acid into the esophagus, which can cause burning substernal chest pain (heartburn).
    - Pathophysiology: The reflux of stomach acids and contents into the esophagus.

- Peptic Ulcer Disease: This involves the formation of ulcers in the lining of the stomach or duodenum. It can cause epigastric pain that may radiate to the chest.
    - Pathophysiology: Open sores in the lining of the stomach or duodenum due to gastric acid and bacterial infection.
- Esophageal Rupture (Boerhaave Syndrome): This life-threatening condition involves a perforation of the esophagus, often due to forceful vomiting. It can cause severe, sudden onset of chest pain, often with associated neck pain.
    - Pathophysiology: A perforation of the esophageal wall, usually due to increased intraluminal pressure.
- Cholecystitis: This is an inflammation of the gallbladder, often caused by gallstones. It can cause right upper quadrant pain that may radiate to the chest.
    - Pathophysiology: Inflammation of the gallbladder, often due to gallstones.
- Pancreatitis: This is an inflammation of the pancreas. It can cause severe upper abdominal pain that can radiate to the chest and back.
    - Pathophysiology: Inflammation of the pancreas, usually caused by gallstones or alcohol misuse

Musculoskeletal Chest Pain

- Costochondritis: This is an inflammation of the cartilage connecting the ribs to the breastbone. It is characterized by localized chest pain often worsened by movement or palpation.
    - Pathophysiology: Inflammation of the cartilage connecting the ribs to the sternum.

- Tietze Syndrome: This is similar to costochondritis, but it involves swelling of the affected cartilage, and may be painful to touch.
    - Pathophysiology: Inflammation of the cartilage connecting the rib to the sternum, with associated swelling.
- Rib Fractures: These are breaks in the rib bones, which can result from trauma. They present with localized pain that is worsened by movement or deep inspiration.
    - Pathophysiology: Breaks or cracks in one or more of the ribs.
- Muscle Strain: This involves injury or pain in the muscles of the chest wall, which can result from strenuous activity.
    - Pathophysiology: Damage to the chest wall muscles due to strain or overuse.
- Fibromyalgia: This is a chronic pain condition that can cause widespread musculoskeletal pain, including chest pain.
    - Pathophysiology: Chronic musculoskeletal pain condition.

Psychogenic Chest Pain

- Panic Disorder: This is characterized by sudden episodes of intense fear or discomfort, often accompanied by chest pain, shortness of breath, palpitations, and dizziness.
    - Pathophysiology: Panic attacks with associated physical symptoms.
- Anxiety: Generalized anxiety can manifest with chest pain, often described as tightness or discomfort, along with other symptoms like restlessness and difficulty concentrating.
    - Pathophysiology: Increased muscular tension and autonomic activity.

- Somatic Symptom Disorder: This is a mental health condition that involves having a significant focus on physical symptoms, such as chest pain, which causes distress and impairment.
  - Pathophysiology: Abnormal focus and distress related to physical symptoms.

Other Causes of Chest Pain

- Herpes Zoster (Shingles): This viral infection can cause painful skin rash with localized chest pain along a nerve path.
  - Pathophysiology: Reactivation of varicella zoster virus, resulting in a painful skin rash along the nerve path.
- Cervical Radiculopathy: This involves compression of a nerve in the cervical spine that can cause pain radiating to the chest.
  - Pathophysiology: Compression of a spinal nerve in the cervical spine.
- Mediastinitis: This is an inflammation of the mediastinum (the space in the chest containing the heart and major vessels), often caused by infection.
  - Pathophysiology: Inflammation of the mediastinum, often due to bacterial infections or post-surgical complications.

Diagnostic Approach to Chest Pain

A systematic diagnostic approach involves a combination of history taking, physical exam, and investigations.

- History Taking:
  - Comprehensive Symptom Analysis (as Detailed Above): Onset, location, radiation, character, intensity, aggravating/relieving factors, associated symptoms.

- Risk Factor Assessment: Including age, sex, family history of cardiac disease, smoking status, presence of hypertension, diabetes, hyperlipidemia, and other conditions.
- Past Medical History: including history of cardiac, pulmonary, gastrointestinal, or other relevant conditions.
- Medication History: A list of all medications including over the counter medication, recreational drugs and herbal medications.

- Physical Examination:
    - Cardiovascular Examination: Includes assessment of heart rate, blood pressure, heart sounds, murmurs, and presence of jugular venous distension.
    - Respiratory Examination: Includes auscultation for breath sounds, wheezes, crackles, assessment of respiratory rate and use of accessory muscles.
    - Musculoskeletal Examination: Includes palpation for tenderness over the chest wall and assessment of range of motion.
    - Abdominal Examination: Includes palpation of the abdomen for tenderness, guarding, and organomegaly.
    - Skin Examination: Includes checking for rashes and for signs of shingles.

- Investigations:
    - Electrocardiogram (ECG): This is essential for the evaluation of cardiac chest pain, identifying signs of ischemia, infarction, or arrhythmias.
    - Cardiac Enzymes (Troponin, CK-MB): These blood tests detect myocardial damage and are crucial in diagnosing acute coronary syndromes.
    - Chest X-ray: This imaging study can help identify pulmonary causes of chest pain, such as pneumonia, pneumothorax, or pleural effusion.

- Computed Tomography (CT) Angiography: This imaging modality is useful for diagnosing pulmonary embolism and aortic dissection.
- Echocardiogram: This ultrasound of the heart assesses its structure and function, aiding in the diagnosis of pericarditis, myocarditis, and valvular disease.
- Upper Endoscopy: This involves inserting a camera into the esophagus and stomach, useful in diagnosing gastrointestinal causes of chest pain like esophagitis, peptic ulcer disease, and esophageal rupture.
- Other Investigations: Such as blood work, sputum samples or specific tests tailored to the clinical scenario.

Red Flags in Chest Pain: When to Suspect Life-Threatening Conditions

Certain presenting features and clinical findings should raise immediate concern for potentially life-threatening conditions:

- Severe, crushing chest pain: Especially when associated with diaphoresis (sweating), nausea, or vomiting (suggestive of ACS).
- Sudden onset of severe chest pain radiating to the back: Suggestive of aortic dissection.
- Sharp, pleuritic chest pain with sudden onset of shortness of breath: Can be a sign of pulmonary embolism or pneumothorax.
- Hemodynamic instability (hypotension, tachycardia, altered mental status): Suggestive of a severe cardiac or pulmonary emergency.
- New-onset chest pain in a patient with multiple risk factors for cardiac disease: Can be indicative of ACS.

The presence of these red flags warrants immediate evaluation and potentially emergent intervention.

Comparative Table of Chest Pain Causes

Feature	**Acute Coronary Syndrome (ACS) (Heart Attack/ Angina)**	**Pulmonary Chest Pain (e.g., Pulmonary Embolism, Pleurisy)**	**Gastrointestinal Chest Pain (e.g., GERD, Esophageal Spasm)**	**Musculoskeletal Chest Pain (e.g., Costochondritis, Muscle Strain)**	**Psychogenic Chest Pain (e.g., Panic Attack, Anxiety)**	**Other Causes of Chest Pain (e.g., Aortic Dissection, Pericarditis)**
Pain Description	Crushing, squeezing, tightness, pressure; may radiate	Sharp, stabbing, worse with breathing or coughing	Burning, often behind the breastbone; may feel like food stuck	Aching, localized, may be tender to touch	Variable, can be sharp, stabbing, dull; often non-specific	Variable depending on the cause: tearing (aortic dissection), sharp (pericarditis)
Pain Location	Often central or left-sided, may radiate to arm, jaw, back	Usually lateral (side of the chest), but can be central	Typically, substernal (behind the breastbone)	Localized to the area of injury or inflammation	Variable; can be anywhere in the chest	Variable; central or anterior (pericarditis), tearing (aortic dissection)
Onset	Sudden, often worsening over minutes	Can be sudden (embolism) or gradual (pleurisy)	Can be gradual (GERD) or sudden (spasm)	Typically associated with activity or injury	Sudden or gradual, often triggered by stress/anxiety	Sudden (aortic dissection), gradual (pericarditis)
Aggravating Factors	Exertion, stress; may not be relieved by rest (unstable angina)	Breathing, coughing, deep breaths	Lying down, large meals, certain foods	Movement, pressure, palpation	Stress, anxiety, emotional distress	Movement (pericarditis), high blood pressure (aortic dissection)

Relieving Factors	Rest, nitro-glycerine (for angina)	Rest, pain medication	Antacids, sitting upright, certain medications	Rest, pain medication, heat or cold	Relaxation techniques, breathing exercises, addressing anxiety	Depends on underlying cause: sitting up or leaning forward for pericarditis
Associated Symptoms	Shortness of breath, sweating, nausea, dizziness	Shortness of breath, cough, hemoptysis (coughing up blood)	Heartburn, regurgitation, difficulty swallowing	Local muscle spasm, swelling, bruising	Palpitations, hyperventilation, fear of impending doom	Palpitations, fever, fatigue (pericarditis), tearing sensation with radiation (aortic dissection)
Duration	Minutes to hours	Minutes to days	Minutes to hours	Days to weeks	Minutes to hours	Variable, hours to days
Severity	Severe to moderate; can be life-threatening	Mild to severe; can be life-threatening	Mild to moderate	Mild to moderate	Mild to severe	Variable, can be life-threatening (aortic dissection)
Key Diagnostic Tests	EKG, blood tests (troponin), imaging (angiography)	Chest X-ray, CT scan with contrast, D-dimer	Endoscopy, pH monitoring, upper GI series	Physical exam, sometimes X-ray	Clinical history, ruling out other causes	EKG, Chest X-ray, CT scan, MRI

Clinical Case Studies: Illustrative Examples of Chest Pain Differential Diagnosis

To demonstrate the complexities of chest pain diagnosis, let's consider a few illustrative cases:

- Case 1: A 60-year-old male with a history of hypertension and smoking presents with a 20-minute history of severe, crushing chest pain radiating to the jaw, accompanied by sweating and nausea. ECG shows ST-segment elevation. *Diagnosis: STEMI.*
- Case 2: A 25-year-old female presents with sharp, stabbing chest pain worsened by breathing, accompanied by fever and cough. Chest X-ray shows consolidation in the right lower lung field *Diagnosis: Pneumonia with Pleuritis.*
- Case 3: A 40-year-old female describes a burning sensation in her chest following meals, along with acid reflux and regurgitation. *Diagnosis: GERD.*
- Case 4: A 35-year-old male presents with localized chest pain after a fall, with point tenderness over the anterior chest wall. *Diagnosis: Rib Fracture.*
- Case 5: A 28-year-old female has intermittent chest pain, often accompanied by shortness of breath, palpitations, and dizziness, occurring at random times. She reports feeling intense fear and anxiety with the attacks. *Diagnosis: Panic Disorder.*

These cases illustrate the diverse presentations of chest pain and how the clinical picture, combined with appropriate investigations, leads to diagnosis.

Summary and Key Takeaways

Chest pain is a common and challenging symptom that requires a systematic and careful approach to evaluation. Key takeaways include:

- Chest pain can arise from a variety of sources, including cardiac, pulmonary, musculoskeletal, gastrointestinal, and psychological origins.

- A thorough history including onset, location, radiation, character, intensity, aggravating/relieving factors, and associated symptoms is essential for building a differential diagnosis, along with a detailed physical examination.
- Investigations such as ECG, cardiac enzymes, chest X-ray, CT angiography, and upper endoscopy play a crucial role in identifying the underlying cause.
- Recognizing red flags is essential to identify and manage potentially life-threatening conditions such as acute coronary syndromes, pulmonary embolism, and aortic dissection promptly.

Differential Diagnosis of Heart Failure

Introduction to Heart Failure

Heart failure (HF), a complex and progressive clinical syndrome, occurs when the heart is unable to pump sufficient blood to meet the body's metabolic needs at normal filling pressures, or can do so only at the expense of elevated filling pressures. This seemingly simple definition belies a multifaceted condition with diverse etiologies, varying clinical presentations, and a significant impact on morbidity and mortality. Understanding the nuances of HF, including its classification, epidemiology, and pathophysiology, is paramount for effective diagnosis and management.

Definition and Classification:

Heart failure is not a single disease, but rather a constellation of signs and symptoms arising from impaired cardiac function. It is broadly classified based on left ventricular ejection fraction (LVEF), a measure of the percentage of blood pumped out of the left ventricle with each contraction:

- Heart Failure with Reduced Ejection Fraction (HFrEF): Characterized by a LVEF of ≤ 40%. This is often associated with systolic dysfunction, where the heart muscle has difficulty contracting effectively. This was previously known as systolic heart failure.

- Heart Failure with Preserved Ejection Fraction (HFpEF): Characterized by a LVEF of ≥ 50%. This is associated with diastolic dysfunction, where the heart has difficulty relaxing and filling properly with blood. This was previously known as diastolic heart failure.
- Heart Failure with Mid-Range Ejection Fraction (HFmrEF): Characterized by a LVEF between 41-49%. This is a relatively newer category and is believed to have an overlapping pathophysiology between HFrEF and HFpEF.

Additionally, HF can be classified based on its onset and severity (acute vs. chronic), its functional classification according to the New York Heart Association (NYHA) criteria (ranging from Class I: no limitation of physical activity to Class IV: symptoms at rest), and whether it affects the right or left side of the heart.

Epidemiology:

Heart failure is a major public health concern, affecting millions worldwide. Its prevalence increases with age, and it is a leading cause of hospitalization and mortality, particularly in developed countries. The incidence of HF is also rising due to factors such as an aging population, improved survival rates following myocardial infarction, and increasing prevalence of risk factors such as hypertension and diabetes. HF is the number one cause of hospitalisation worldwide. A significant disparity between the occurrence of HFrEF and HFpEF exists between men and women, with men being more likely to have HFrEF and women HFpEF. The prevalence of both increases exponentially as people age.

Pathophysiology of Heart Failure

The underlying pathophysiology of heart failure is complex and multifactorial, involving a cascade of cellular, molecular, and neurohumoral mechanisms. The cardinal features are systolic and diastolic dysfunction leading to reduced cardiac output and compensatory structural adaptations of the heart.

Systolic Dysfunction:

Systolic dysfunction, predominantly seen in HFrEF, arises from decreased myocardial contractility. This is often a result of:

- Myocardial Damage: Ischemic heart disease (myocardial infarction), cardiomyopathies, and myocarditis can damage or weaken heart muscle cells, impairing their ability to contract.
- Volume Overload: Chronic conditions such as valvular regurgitation or intracardiac shunts can lead to ventricular dilation (enlargement) which may lead to impaired contractility.
- Pressure Overload: Conditions like hypertension or aortic stenosis increase workload on the heart and might result in systolic dysfunction.

Diastolic Dysfunction:

Diastolic dysfunction, commonly associated with HFpEF, is characterized by impaired ventricular relaxation and filling. This may not reduce the ejection fraction but reduces overall stroke volume by reducing end diastolic volume. The major mechanisms involved are:

- Increased Myocardial Stiffness: Conditions like hypertension, hypertrophic cardiomyopathy, and infiltrative diseases (e.g., amyloidosis) can lead to increased stiffness of the left ventricle and reduce its compliance.
- Impaired Myocardial Relaxation: Dysfunction of calcium handling within heart muscle cells can disrupt the normal relaxation process.
- Ventricular Hypertrophy: Increased muscle mass in the heart can lead to elevated filling pressures and diastolic dysfunction.

Neurohumoral Activation:

In response to the reduced cardiac output and/or increased filling pressures, the neurohumoral systems of the body become activated. This initially serves as a compensatory mechanism to maintain cardiac output and blood pressure, but chronically these systems can become detrimental:

- Sympathetic Nervous System (SNS): Increased SNS activity leads to elevated heart rate and vasoconstriction, which may increase heart workload.
- Renin-Angiotensin-Aldosterone System (RAAS): RAAS activation leads to sodium and water retention, increasing the circulating blood volume and cardiac preload.
- Natriuretic Peptides: Release of natriuretic peptides (BNP, ANP) in attempt to reduce circulating blood volume, and act as vasodilators.

Key Presenting Features of Heart Failure

The clinical manifestation of HF is highly variable, depending on the underlying cause, the chronicity of the condition, and the degree of cardiac dysfunction. The most common presenting symptoms of heart failure include:

- Dyspnea (Shortness of Breath): Dyspnea is often the most common complaint, arising from pulmonary congestion due to increased pressure in the pulmonary vasculature.
    - Exertional Dyspnea: Breathlessness during physical activity, is a hallmark of heart failure.
    - Orthopnea: Breathlessness when lying flat, relieved by sitting or standing.
    - Paroxysmal Nocturnal Dyspnea (PND): Sudden episodes of severe breathlessness, awakening the patient from sleep.
- Fatigue: A consequence of reduced cardiac output and inadequate tissue perfusion and metabolic changes in the muscle.

- Edema: Swelling, especially in the lower legs, ankles, and feet, resulting from fluid retention due to elevated venous pressures. It may be pitting or non-pitting.
- Other Symptoms: Patients may also experience cough (especially at night), decreased appetite or nausea, weight gain, palpitations, and cognitive impairment.

Differential Diagnosis of Heart Failure

While the presenting features of HF are often suggestive, many other conditions can mimic its signs and symptoms. A comprehensive differential diagnosis is crucial to ensure appropriate management.

Cardiac Causes of Heart Failure:

- Ischemic Heart Disease (Coronary Artery Disease, Myocardial Infarction): Coronary artery disease (CAD) and its sequelae are the single most common cause of HF worldwide, and is more likely to result in systolic dysfunction. Myocardial infarction (MI) leads to loss of viable heart muscle, reducing contractile function.
    - Diagnosis: History of chest pain, ECG changes, elevated cardiac biomarkers (troponin), and coronary angiography.
- Valvular Heart Disease (Aortic Stenosis, Mitral Regurgitation, etc.): Valvular abnormalities disrupt the normal flow of blood through the heart, leading to volume and/or pressure overload. They can cause either systolic or diastolic dysfunction depending on the issue.
    - Diagnosis: Cardiac auscultation revealing heart murmurs, echocardiography to visualize valve morphology and function.
- Cardiomyopathies (Dilated, Hypertrophic, Restrictive): Cardiomyopathies are diseases of the heart muscle itself. They can lead to abnormal contraction or relaxation of the heart.

  - Dilated Cardiomyopathy: Characterized by enlargement of the heart chambers which can lead to both systolic and diastolic dysfunction.
  - Hypertrophic Cardiomyopathy: Characterized by thickening of the heart muscle, often the septum. This can lead to diastolic dysfunction and is a leading cause of sudden cardiac death.
  - Restrictive Cardiomyopathy: Characterized by stiffening of the heart muscle, limiting filling capacity therefore resulting in diastolic dysfunction.
  - Diagnosis: Echocardiography, cardiac MRI, genetic testing where applicable.

- Hypertension-Related Heart Failure: Chronic, uncontrolled hypertension forces the heart to work harder, ultimately leading to left ventricular hypertrophy and diastolic dysfunction and can eventually progress to systolic dysfunction.

  - Diagnosis: History of hypertension, elevated blood pressure findings, and evidence of left ventricular hypertrophy on ECG or echocardiography.

- Arrhythmias (Atrial Fibrillation, Tachycardia-Mediated Cardiomyopathy): Sustained arrhythmias can lead to atrial fibrillation can lead to both systolic and diastolic heart failure over time. Also, tachycardia may lead to reduced diastolic filling and over a longer period of time, tachycardia induced cardiomyopathy.
- Diagnosis: ECG abnormalities, Holter monitoring, Electrophysiology studies.
- Congenital Heart Disease: Structural abnormalities present at birth can result in abnormal blood flow and pressure overload, eventually leading to heart failure.

  - Diagnosis: Childhood history, cardiac auscultation, echocardiography, MRI.

- Pericardial Disease (Constrictive Pericarditis, Cardiac Tamponade): Conditions affecting the pericardium (sac surrounding the heart) can restrict cardiac filling and output.
  - Constrictive Pericarditis: Inflammation of the pericardium leads to scarring restricting filling of the heart.
  - Cardiac Tamponade: Accumulation of fluid in the pericardial space compresses the heart and leads to impaired filling.
  - Diagnosis: Specific ECG changes, echocardiography, CT/MRI, clinical signs such as pulsus paradoxus and Kussmaul's sign.

- Myocarditis and Inflammatory Cardiomyopathies: Inflammation of the heart muscle, often resulting from viral infections or autoimmune diseases can impair systolic function and may result in cardiomyopathy.
  - Diagnosis: Elevated inflammatory markers, cardiac MRI, endomyocardial biopsy.

- Endocrine Disorders (Hyperthyroidism, Hypothyroidism, Pheochromocytoma): Endocrine disorders can affect cardiac function both directly and indirectly.
  - Hyperthyroidism: Elevated thyroid hormones increase heart rate and contractility, which can lead to high-output heart failure.
  - Hypothyroidism: Low thyroid hormone levels may contribute to cardiac dysfunction, heart rate is typically decreased, leading to low output heart failure.
  - Pheochromocytoma: Catecholamine-secreting tumors can lead to elevated heart rate, blood pressure, and cardiomyopathy.
  - Diagnosis: Thyroid function tests, catecholamine levels, imaging studies as indicated.

- Drug-Induced Cardiomyopathy (Chemotherapy, Alcohol, Cocaine): Certain drugs and substances can cause damage to the heart muscle, leading to cardiomyopathy and heart failure.
    - Diagnosis: History of substance use and/or specific medication use, echocardiography.

Non-Cardiac Causes Mimicking Heart Failure:

- Pulmonary Hypertension: Elevated pressure in the pulmonary arteries can lead to right-sided heart failure or mimic left-sided failure presenting with dyspnea, fatigue and edema. In primary pulmonary hypertension the arteries themselves are dysfunctional and in secondary it is caused by an external cause like COPD, or chronic thromboembolic pulmonary disease.
    - Diagnosis: Elevated pulmonary artery pressures on echocardiography, right heart catheterization.
- Pulmonary Embolism: Sudden blockage of a pulmonary artery by a blood clot can lead to acute right-sided heart overload and dyspnea, mimicking acute heart failure and can also lead to long term pulmonary hypertension.
    - Diagnosis: CT pulmonary angiogram, D-dimer test, V/Q scan.
- Chronic Obstructive Pulmonary Disease (COPD): Airflow limitation and hyperinflation in COPD can lead to dyspnea, chronic cough, and can eventually result in right sided heart failure.
    - Diagnosis: History of smoking, pulmonary function tests.
- Asthma: Airway inflammation and bronchoconstriction in asthma can cause dyspnea and wheezing, potentially mimicking some features of heart failure.
    - Diagnosis: History of asthma, pulmonary function tests improved with bronchodilators, clinical response to treatment.

- Obesity-Related Dyspnea: Obese individuals may experience dyspnea, especially with exertion, due to mechanical factors, and restrictive lung disease.
    - Diagnosis: Physical examination and correlation with BMI.
- Renal Failure with Fluid Overload: Impaired kidney function leads to fluid retention, increased blood volume, and electrolyte imbalances, which can result in symptoms similar to heart failure with edema and dyspnea.
    - Diagnosis: Elevated creatinine and BUN, electrolyte imbalances, renal ultrasound.
- Liver Cirrhosis with Fluid Overload: Liver dysfunction can cause fluid retention (ascites, edema) due to hypoalbuminemia and portal hypertension which can mimic signs of heart failure. The circulatory dysfunction in cirrhosis may also cause heart failure.
    - Diagnosis: Elevated liver enzymes, abnormal bilirubin levels, clinical signs of liver disease.
- Anemia: Severe anemia can lead to high output heart failure due to increased cardiac demand to maintain oxygen delivery, resulting in dyspnea and fatigue.
    - Diagnosis: Complete blood count revealing low haemoglobin.
- Hypervolemia from Other Causes (e.g., Excessive Intravenous Fluids): Iatrogenic (medically induced) fluid overload can cause similar signs and symptoms as heart failure including edema, dyspnea, and weight gain.
    - Diagnosis: Clinical history and response to treatment.

Diagnostic Approach to Heart Failure

A systematic approach is essential for accurately diagnosing heart failure and differentiating it from other conditions. It typically entails a combination of history taking, physical examination, and diagnostic investigations.

History Taking:

A detailed history of symptoms, risk factors, co-morbidities, and medication use helps to narrow down the differential diagnosis. Key elements include:

- Nature and Duration of Symptoms: Onset, triggers, aggravating and relieving factors of dyspnea, fatigue, edema.
- Past Medical History: Including history of ischemic heart disease, hypertension, diabetes, valvular disease, arrhythmias, and cardiomyopathies.
- Risk Factors: Smoking, obesity, family history of heart disease.
- Co-Morbidities: Renal disease, liver disease, lung disease, and any other relevant medical conditions.
- Medication History: Current and past medications, including drugs that may have cardiotoxic effects.
- Social History: Including alcohol intake, drug use, and occupation.

Physical Examination:

A thorough physical examination is crucial to evaluate the hemodynamic status and detect signs suggestive of heart failure:

- Cardiovascular Examination: Heart rate, rhythm (regular/irregular), heart sounds (murmurs, gallops). Jugular venous pressure (JVP), assessing for elevation which may indicate fluid overload or right sided heart failure.
- Respiratory Examination: Respiratory rate, breath sounds (rales/crackles, wheezes), oxygen saturation.
- Fluid Status Assessment: Checking for peripheral edema (location, pitting vs. non-pitting), ascites, and weight gain.
- Other Relevant Findings: Cyanosis, hepatomegaly (enlarged liver), abdominal tenderness.
- General appearance and cachexia (muscle wasting).

Investigations:

Laboratory tests and imaging studies are vital for confirming the diagnosis of heart failure, determining the specific cause, and assessing the severity of the condition.

- Electrocardiogram (ECG): Can identify arrhythmias, ischemic changes, left ventricular hypertrophy, and other abnormalities that may contribute to heart failure.
- Chest X-ray: Can reveal cardiomegaly, pulmonary congestion, pleural effusions, and other pulmonary abnormalities.
- Echocardiogram: The most important imaging modality for diagnosing and characterizing heart failure. It assesses the LVEF, chamber size, wall motion abnormalities, valvular function, and diastolic function.
- Brain Natriuretic Peptide (BNP) or NT-proBNP: Elevated levels of these markers suggest increased ventricular wall stress and can be used as a diagnostic and prognostic tool.
- Renal Function Tests: Serum creatinine, blood urea nitrogen (BUN), and estimated glomerular filtration rate (eGFR) to evaluate renal function and its contribution to fluid overload.
- Liver Function Tests: Alanine transaminase (ALT), aspartate transaminase (AST), alkaline phosphatase, bilirubin levels, albumin to assess for liver disease as a possible cause.
- Thyroid Function Tests: Thyroid stimulating hormone (TSH) and thyroid hormones (T3, T4) to assess for thyroid dysfunction as a potential underlying cause.
- Other Investigations (as needed): Complete blood count, coagulation studies, electrolyte levels, arterial blood gas, stress testing, coronary angiography, cardiac MRI or CT.

Feature	Heart Failure with Reduced Ejection Fraction (HFrEF)	Heart Failure with Preserved Ejection Fraction (HFpEF)	Stage A (At Risk)	Stage B (Pre-HF)	Stage C (Symptomatic)	Stage D (Advanced)
Primary Problem	Weakened pumping ability; heart muscle can't contract strongly.	Heart muscle contracts normally, but the heart can't relax properly.	Risk factors present, no structural heart disease.	Structural heart disease present, no symptoms.	Current or past symptoms of heart failure.	Severe symptoms despite optimal treatment.
Ejection Fraction (EF)	Reduced, typically 40% or less.	Normal or nearly normal, typically 50% or more.	Not applicable	Not applicable	Can be reduced or preserved	Reduced or preserved, usually severely reduced.
Heart Muscle	Enlarged, weakened.	Stiff, thickened.	Normal	May have early changes	Structural changes are present	Significant damage, often enlarged.
Causes	Coronary artery disease, heart attack, cardiomyopathy, valve problems.	High blood pressure, diabetes, older age, obesity, restrictive cardiomyopathy.	High blood pressure, diabetes, family history, substance abuse, etc.	Known heart conditions like prior heart attack, valve disease.	Progress of previous stages	Refractory to treatment, severe underlying disease

Common Symptoms	Fatigue, shortness of breath, swelling in legs and ankles.	Fatigue, shortness of breath, difficulty with activity.	No symptoms	Usually no symptoms.	Same as HFrEF and HFpEF	Severe fatigue, shortness of breath even at rest, require specialized interventions.
Treatment Focuses	Medications to improve pumping function, address underlying conditions, lifestyle changes.	Medications to manage blood pressure and other comorbidities, lifestyle changes.	Lifestyle modifications to address risk factors	Address underlying issues, regular monitoring	Medications based on EF, address underlying issues, lifestyle changes	Advanced therapies, palliative care, transplant
Prognosis	Can be variable, depends on severity, often responds to treatment.	Can be variable, may be more difficult to treat.	Prevention is key	Prevent progression to symptomatic HF	Management of symptoms & prevent worsening	Often poor, specialized care required

Diagnostic Criteria for Heart Failure

The diagnosis of heart failure relies on the integration of clinical findings and echocardiographic data:

- Symptoms Consistent with Heart Failure: Dyspnea, fatigue, edema, orthopnea, paroxysmal nocturnal dyspnea.
- Echocardiographic Evidence of Cardiac Dysfunction: Reduced LVEF in HFrEF or evidence of diastolic dysfunction in HFpEF.
- Elevated BNP or NT-proBNP levels: Help to add to the probability of a cardiac cause of dyspnea.

Not all 3 points need to be present to make the diagnosis of heart failure.

Clinical Case Studies: Illustrative Examples of Heart Failure Differential Diagnosis

Let's explore a few hypothetical cases to demonstrate how the differential diagnosis of heart failure is approached in clinical practice:

Case 1: 65-year-old Male with Acute Dyspnea

- History: Presents to the emergency department with severe dyspnea, orthopnea, and paroxysmal nocturnal dyspnea. He has a history of hypertension and type 2 diabetes. No chest pain.
- Physical Examination: Tachycardia, bibasilar crackles, elevated JVP, and pitting edema in the lower extremities.
- ECG: Sinus tachycardia, left ventricular hypertrophy.
- Chest X-ray: Cardiomegaly, pulmonary congestion.
- BNP: Significantly elevated.
- Echocardiogram: Reduced LVEF (35%), dilated left ventricle, mitral regurgitation.
- Differential: This case is highly suggestive of acute decompensated heart failure secondary to ischemic heart disease and/or hypertension. A thorough evaluation, including coronary

angiography, should be done to assess for myocardial ischemia. Pulmonary embolism would also remain in the differential.

Case 2: 72-year-old Female with Exertional Dyspnea

- History: Gradual onset of exertional dyspnea over several months. She has a history of hypertension and hyperlipidemia. Complains of fatigue. No chest pain and no significant edema.
- Physical Examination: Normal heart sounds, no murmurs, mild bibasilar crackles, normal JVP, and no edema.
- ECG: Normal sinus rhythm, left ventricular hypertrophy.
- Chest X-ray: Mild cardiomegaly, no acute pulmonary congestion.
- BNP: Mildly elevated.
- Echocardiogram: Normal LVEF (60%), left ventricular hypertrophy, mild diastolic dysfunction.
- Differential: This case is suggestive of HFpEF due to hypertension. Further investigation for underlying causes of diastolic dysfunction is needed. Differential diagnoses would include restrictive cardiomyopathy, pericardial disease or an alternative cause for the dyspnea.

Case 3: 50-year-old Male with Chronic Dyspnea and Cough

- History: Chronic dyspnea and chronic cough, with frequent exacerbations. History of smoking.
- Physical Examination: Increased anteroposterior diameter, hyperresonance to percussion, wheezes on auscultation.
- ECG: Sinus tachycardia, right ventricular hypertrophy.
- Chest X-ray: Hyperinflation of the lungs, flattened hemidiaphragms.
- BNP: Mildly elevated.
- Echocardiogram: Normal LVEF (55%), possible right ventricular dysfunction but otherwise normal heart.
- Differential: This case is more consistent with COPD, not heart failure. However, he may have secondary pulmonary hypertension

due to COPD contributing to dyspnea. A pulmonary function test would help confirm diagnosis.

Summary and Key Takeaways

The differential diagnosis of heart failure is complex and requires a thorough understanding of its pathophysiology, clinical presentations, and the various cardiac and non-cardiac conditions that can mimic its signs and symptoms. A systematic approach using a focused history, physical examination, and carefully chosen diagnostic investigations is crucial. Key takeaways include:

- Heart failure is a heterogeneous syndrome with varied etiologies and clinical manifestations.
- Distinguishing between HFrEF and HFpEF is essential for guiding management.
- Non-cardiac causes of dyspnea and edema must always be considered.
- A combination of clinical data, ECG, chest x-ray, echocardiography, and BNP levels forms the basis for accurate diagnosis.
- Clinical case studies illustrate the practical application of differential diagnostic thinking.
- Early and accurate diagnosis is essential for timely intervention and improved patient outcomes.

Bibliography

(A comprehensive bibliography would include a list of relevant textbooks, guidelines and journal articles - to list these here may be cumbersome so a general statement will be made)

This article is based on established medical knowledge and guidelines on the diagnosis and management of heart failure. For a comprehensive list of references please refer to relevant cardiology guidelines, textbooks and publications from reputable sources.

This expanded article provides a robust foundation for understanding the differential diagnosis of heart failure. It combines theoretical knowledge with practical clinical considerations and illustrative case studies, while maintaining an accessible style that should benefit a wide range of readers, from medical students to practitioners.

Differential Diagnosis of Arterial Hypertension

Introduction to Arterial Hypertension

Arterial hypertension, commonly referred to as high blood pressure, is a prevalent and significant global health concern. It is characterized by a sustained elevation of arterial blood pressure above the normal range. Blood pressure, measured in millimetres of mercury (mmHg), is the force exerted by circulating blood against the walls of blood vessels. It is expressed as two numbers: systolic pressure (the pressure when the heart contracts) and diastolic pressure (the pressure when the heart relaxes). A blood pressure reading is typically represented as systolic pressure over diastolic pressure (e.g., 120/80 mmHg).

Based on guidelines from various organizations, including the American Heart Association (AHA) and the European Society of Cardiology (ESC), hypertension is generally defined as a systolic blood pressure of 130 mmHg or higher, or a diastolic blood pressure of 80 mmHg or higher. However, these guidelines are subject to ongoing revisions based on the latest research and clinical evidence.

Classification of Hypertension

Hypertension is classified into several stages based on blood pressure readings:

1. Normal Blood Pressure: Less than 120/80 mmHg.
2. Elevated Blood Pressure: Systolic pressure between 120-129 mmHg and diastolic pressure less than 80 mmHg.
3. Stage 1 Hypertension: Systolic pressure between 130-139 mmHg or diastolic pressure between 80-89 mmHg.

4. Stage 2 Hypertension: Systolic pressure of 140 mmHg or higher, or diastolic pressure of 90 mmHg or higher.
5. Hypertensive Crisis: Systolic blood pressure over 180 mmHg or diastolic blood pressure over 120 mmHg, often requiring immediate medical intervention.

Further, hypertension can be categorized as either primary (essential) or secondary hypertension based on its etiology.

Prevalence of Hypertension

Hypertension is a global public health issue, affecting a substantial portion of the adult population. Estimates vary, but it is believed that over a billion individuals worldwide have hypertension. Prevalence increases with age, and it affects men and women differently at various age groups. Factors contributing to the high prevalence include aging populations, unhealthy lifestyles (including poor diet and lack of physical activity), and increased stress. The prevalence also varies geographically, with higher rates observed in some regions and populations. It is crucial to understand the significant impact of uncontrolled hypertension, as it is a major risk factor for cardiovascular diseases (such as heart attack and stroke), kidney disease, and other health complications. These consequences place a significant burden on healthcare systems worldwide. Therefore, early detection, treatment, and management of hypertension are imperative for public health improvement.

Pathophysiology of Arterial Hypertension

Understanding the mechanisms behind hypertension is crucial for effective management. The pathophysiology is complex, involving several interacting systems and factors that influence the regulation of blood pressure. In general, blood pressure is determined by two main factors: cardiac output (the amount of blood pumped by the heart per minute) and peripheral vascular resistance (the resistance to blood flow in the arteries).

Primary (Essential) Hypertension

Primary or essential hypertension constitutes approximately 90-95% of all cases of hypertension. Its etiology is multifactorial, with genetic predisposition, lifestyle choices, and environmental factors playing crucial roles.

1. Genetic Factors: Family history is a significant risk factor, suggesting a strong genetic component. Research has identified numerous genes that are associated with increased susceptibility to hypertension. These genes often regulate processes such as the renin-angiotensin-aldosterone system (RAAS), sodium handling, and vascular smooth muscle contraction.
2. Lifestyle factors: These include:
    - Dietary Factors: High sodium intake, low potassium intake, and consumption of processed foods contribute to increased blood pressure.
    - Lack of Physical Activity: Sedentary lifestyles contribute to weight gain which is linked with hypertension.
    - Obesity: An increased body mass index (BMI) and excess adiposity are directly associated with high blood pressure, due to increased cardiac output and activation of RAAS.
    - Excessive Alcohol Consumption: Heavy drinking can elevate blood pressure by various mechanisms, including increased sympathetic nervous system activity and RAAS activation.
    - Smoking: Nicotine and other toxins in tobacco products damage the blood vessels and increase blood pressure.
    - Stress: Chronic stress may lead to hypertension through the activation of the sympathetic nervous system and the hypothalamic-pituitary-adrenal (HPA) axis.
3. Environmental Factors: Exposure to toxins and certain chemicals can contribute to the development of hypertension. Environmental pollution also increases stress levels and thereby contributing to hypertension.

Secondary Hypertension

Secondary hypertension accounts for only 5-10% of hypertension cases and is caused by an identifiable underlying medical condition. Treating the underlying cause is often essential in managing secondary hypertension.

Mechanisms of Blood Pressure Regulation

Blood pressure is tightly regulated by several intricate mechanisms, including neural, hormonal, and renal systems.

1. Neural Control: The sympathetic and parasympathetic nervous systems exert significant control over blood pressure. The sympathetic nervous system increases heart rate and constricts blood vessels, thus elevating blood pressure. The parasympathetic system has the opposite effect, lowering heart rate and promoting vasodilation.
2. Hormonal Regulation: Several hormones, including the RAAS, play crucial roles in long-term blood pressure regulation. Renin, produced by the kidneys, initiates the RAAS cascade, which leads to vasoconstriction and increased sodium and water retention, thus increasing blood pressure. Adrenaline and noradrenaline, produced by the adrenal glands, cause an increase in heart rate and vasoconstriction, leading to a rise in blood pressure.
3. Renal Control: The kidneys play a pivotal role in long-term blood pressure regulation through the control of sodium and water balance. Kidneys regulate blood volume through excretion or retention of water and sodium which influences blood pressure directly.
4. Endothelial Factors: The endothelium, a layer of cells lining blood vessels, produces various substances that influence vascular tone. Endothelial dysfunction, seen in conditions like atherosclerosis, leads to impaired vasodilation and contributes to hypertension.

Key Presenting Features of Arterial Hypertension

Arterial hypertension is often called the “silent killer” because it is frequently asymptomatic, especially in its early stages. Many individuals are unaware that they have hypertension until a routine check-up reveals the condition, or a complication arises. However, when symptoms do appear they can include:

1. Often Asymptomatic: The most common characteristic of hypertension is its lack of noticeable symptoms. Many individuals live for years with elevated blood pressure without any overt signs.
2. Headache: Especially a throbbing or pulsatile headache, is often associated with hypertension, especially when the blood pressure is very high.
3. Dizziness: Dizziness or light headedness may occur, although these symptoms are less specific and can be caused by various other conditions.
4. Blurred Vision: Visual disturbances, such as blurred or double vision, may result from damage to retinal blood vessels secondary to hypertension.
5. Epistaxis (Severe Hypertension): Nosebleeds are rare symptoms of hypertension and more common with severe hypertension or hypertensive emergencies.
6. Other Rare Symptoms: Some patients experiencing significant hypertension might complain of tinnitus (ringing in the ears), shortness of breath, chest pain or even fatigue. These symptoms can be due to target organ damage caused by sustained elevated blood pressure.

Differential Diagnosis of Arterial Hypertension

The differential diagnosis of arterial hypertension involves distinguishing between primary and various secondary forms. The approach is based on understanding the underlying pathological mechanisms of these conditions.

Essential (Primary) Hypertension

Essential hypertension is diagnosed when no specific underlying cause is found and typically is a diagnosis of exclusion. The multifactorial etiology of this condition makes identifying a singular cause challenging. Essential hypertension is diagnosed by ruling out various secondary causes and risk factors.

Secondary Hypertension

Secondary hypertension results from an identified underlying medical condition. It often presents with certain clues that can lead to the diagnosis.

Renal Causes

The kidneys are vital in blood pressure regulation; thus, conditions affecting the kidneys can frequently lead to secondary hypertension. Common renal causes include:

1. Renal Artery Stenosis: Narrowing of one or both renal arteries reduces blood flow to the kidneys. In response, renin is released, activating the RAAS, resulting in increased vasoconstriction and sodium retention, thus leading to hypertension. Renal artery stenosis can be caused by atherosclerosis in older adults and less commonly, fibromuscular dysplasia in younger individuals.
2. Chronic Kidney Disease (CKD): Conditions such as glomerulonephritis and polycystic kidney disease (PKD) can disrupt renal function, leading to fluid and electrolyte imbalances and thereby hypertension. Impaired kidney function due to CKD results in reduced excretion of sodium and water, leading to volume overload and increased blood pressure.
3. Renovascular Hypertension: This term encompasses hypertension caused by various pathologies affecting the renal arteries, including stenosis or other vasculopathies. It can be a primary cause or a consequence of CKD.

4. Renin-Producing Tumors: These rare tumors, usually arising from the juxtaglomerular cells of the kidney, overproduce renin, leading to severe hypertension. They must be kept in mind in cases with resistant hypertension.

Endocrine Causes

Dysfunction of the endocrine system can cause several hormonal imbalances that can lead to secondary hypertension:

1. Primary Aldosteronism (Conn's Syndrome): Characterized by the overproduction of aldosterone by the adrenal glands, leading to sodium retention and potassium loss. This results in increased blood volume and elevated blood pressure. Primary Aldosteronism is a common cause of secondary hypertension.
2. Cushing's Syndrome: Results from chronic exposure to high levels of cortisol. Cortisol has mineralocorticoid effect, and in high levels, will exert that effect, leading to fluid and sodium retention and therefore hypertension. Cushing's syndrome is often caused by exogenous steroids or adrenal or pituitary tumors.
3. Pheochromocytoma: A rare tumor of the adrenal glands that produces excessive amounts of catecholamines (adrenaline and noradrenaline). These hormones lead to marked vasoconstriction and elevated blood pressure, often with episodic hypertensive crises, characterized by severe headache, palpitations, and sweating.
4. Hyperthyroidism: Excessive thyroid hormone levels increase heart rate and cardiac output, thereby elevating systolic blood pressure. Diastolic blood pressure is usually normal or low in hyperthyroidism.
5. Acromegaly: A condition caused by excessive growth hormone, leading to increased tissue mass and elevated blood pressure. This frequently presents with other features such as enlarged hands and feet, and facial dysmorphism.

6. Hyperparathyroidism: High levels of parathyroid hormone can lead to hypercalcemia, which can interfere with vascular smooth muscle contraction and contribute to hypertension, among its other consequences.

Cardiovascular Causes

Several cardiovascular conditions can lead to secondary hypertension.

1. Coarctation of the Aorta: A congenital condition characterized by narrowing of the aorta, which decreases blood flow to the lower body and increases blood pressure in the upper body. Coarctation often manifests with a difference in blood pressure between the upper and lower extremities and is often identified in childhood or adolescence.
2. Aortic Regurgitation: Inability of the aortic valve to close properly, leading to backflow of blood to the left ventricle. This increases systolic blood pressure and decreases diastolic blood pressure. This is usually a late finding with aortic regurgitation.
3. Increased Intracranial Pressure: conditions such as tumors or hemorrhage can cause increased intracranial pressure which leads to a condition called Cushing's reflex. This reflex presents with hypertension, bradycardia and irregular breathing.

Medication-Induced Hypertension

Several medications can cause or exacerbate hypertension, which should always be considered as a potential cause of elevated blood pressure:

1. Nonsteroidal Anti-inflammatory Drugs (NSAIDs): These drugs can cause sodium and fluid retention, increasing blood pressure. They are commonly used for pain relief but often underappreciated as cause of hypertension
2. Oral Contraceptives: Hormonal contraceptives can increase blood pressure due to the effects of estrogen and progestin on the renin-angiotensin system.

3. Glucocorticoids: Long-term or high-dose glucocorticoid use can cause hypertension, mainly through mineralocorticoid effects, like in Cushing's syndrome
4. Decongestants: These drugs, containing sympathetic agonists like pseudoephedrine, can increase heart rate and blood pressure.
5. Erythropoietin: This medication, used to stimulate red blood cell production, can cause hypertension, potentially due to its effects on blood viscosity and vascular tone.
6. Monoamine Oxidase Inhibitors (MAOIs): While less common now, MAOIs used as antidepressants can cause a hypertensive crisis, especially when taken with certain foods.
7. Some Herbal Supplements: Some herbal and over-the-counter supplements can interact with medications or have intrinsic effects that cause hypertension.

Sleep Apnea

1. Obstructive Sleep Apnea: Repeated episodes of upper airway obstruction during sleep cause hypoxia and sympathetic activation, leading to hypertension. Sleep apnea is an underdiagnosed and undertreated condition and its role in hypertension is often overlooked.

Pregnancy-Related Hypertension

1. Preeclampsia: A condition during pregnancy characterized by new-onset hypertension and proteinuria (protein in the urine). It can progress to seizures called eclampsia. Pregnancy-related hypertension poses a serious risk to both the mother and the fetus and requires careful management.

Rare Causes

1. Carcinoid Syndrome: Caused by carcinoid tumors that secrete vasoactive substances leading to both hypertension and hypotension, with other features such as flushing, diarrhea and wheezing episodes.

2. Lead Poisoning: Chronic lead exposure can impair renal function, activate RAAS, and also contribute to hypertension.

Diagnostic Approach to Arterial Hypertension

A systematic approach is vital when evaluating a patient with hypertension. The process involves a detailed history, thorough physical examination, and judicious use of investigations to either confirm the diagnosis or identify the underlying cause.

History Taking

A careful medical history can provide valuable clues:

1. Family History: A detailed family history may reveal genetic predisposition to hypertension or predisposing conditions like renal disease or thyroid disease. Family history of early-onset hypertension is also important since essential hypertension starts earlier in life.
2. Lifestyle Factors: Inquiry about diet, exercise habits, smoking, alcohol, and stress levels can provide critical insights into modifiable risk factors for hypertension.
3. Medications: It is critical to obtain a comprehensive list of medications, both prescription and over-the-counter, including herbal and supplements, to identify a potential drug-induced cause of hypertension.
4. Symptoms Suggestive of Secondary Hypertension: Certain symptoms could suggest a secondary cause. For example, a patient with episodic headaches, sweating, and palpitations might have pheochromocytoma; a patient with snoring and daytime sleepiness might have obstructive sleep apnea; a patient with muscle weakness with hypertension might have hyperaldosteronism.
5. Past Medical History: Asking about past medical conditions, especially kidney diseases, thyroid diseases or previous strokes or heart attacks may elucidate the cause of hypertension.

Physical Examination

A thorough physical examination is crucial in diagnosing and assessing the impact of hypertension

1. Blood Pressure Measurement: Accurate measurements of blood pressure, using a properly sized cuff, in both arms (and sometimes legs) are essential to confirm the diagnosis and aid in monitoring it. Three blood pressure measurements should be taken in a first visit to establish baseline.
2. Fundoscopic Examination: Examination of the retina using an ophthalmoscope can reveal signs of hypertensive retinopathy such as arterio-venous nicking, exudates, hemorrhages, and in very advanced stages, papilledema.
3. Cardiovascular Examination: This includes assessment for cardiomegaly, murmurs, and arrhythmias. Examination for peripheral edema and the presence of bruits should also be noted because they are associated with congestive heart failure and peripheral artery disease respectively.
4. Abdominal Examination: Checking for renal masses, bruits, or other abdominal abnormalities may indicate renal causes of hypertension.
5. Neurological Examination: A neurological examination is done to identify any neurological deficits that may be associated with long-standing hypertension or cerebrovascular disease.
6. Other Examinations: Examination of neck for thyroid enlargement might reveal thyroid disorders that are indirectly causing hypertension.

Investigations

When hypertension is detected, certain investigations will help in establishing its etiology.

1. Urinalysis: Tests for protein, red blood cells, and other abnormalities, essential for assessing renal involvement.

2. Serum Electrolytes: Measures of sodium, potassium, chloride, and bicarbonate help assess fluid balance and can point towards primary aldosteronism.
3. Renal Function Tests: Serum creatinine, BUN, and eGFR help evaluate kidney function, crucial for detecting CKD.
4. Thyroid Function Tests: TSH, T3, and T4 levels can identify hypo/hyperthyroidism.
5. Plasma Renin and Aldosterone Levels: Measuring these hormones helps identify hyperaldosteronism and some other causes of secondary hypertension.
6. 24-Hour Urinary Catecholamines/Metanephrines: These measures are important in diagnosing pheochromocytoma.
7. Renal Ultrasound/Doppler: Imaging of the kidneys to evaluate the renal arteries and kidney parenchyma for stenosis or structural abnormalities.
8. CT/MRI of Adrenal Glands: Imaging of the adrenal glands can help detect adrenal tumors, including those that produce excessive aldosterone or catecholamines.

Screening for Secondary Hypertension

Screening for secondary hypertension is essential, especially in the following circumstances:

1. Early Onset of Hypertension (before age of 30): Hypertension developing at a young age often suggests a secondary cause.
2. Resistant Hypertension: When hypertension is refractory to three or more antihypertensive medications, considering secondary causes is crucial.
3. Sudden Onset/Worsening of Hypertension: A sudden change in blood pressure control should prompt investigation for a secondary cause.
4. Clinical Clues: Specific symptoms or physical findings suggestive of secondary hypertension should lead to further screening.

5. Significant Hypokalemia: Low serum potassium levels in the presence of high blood pressure is highly suggestive of hyperaldosteronism
6. Marked difference in arm and leg blood pressure: Should raise the suspicion for coarctation of the aorta.
7. Algorithms for Screening: Several algorithms are available to help guide the appropriate investigations in a logical sequence. Initial tests might include urinalysis, serum electrolytes, renal function tests, and thyroid function tests. Based on these results, further investigations like renin/aldosterone levels, urinary catecholamines, renal doppler, or adrenal imaging, may be indicated.

Comparative Summary of Arterial Hypertension

The following table presents a simplified comparison of common classifications of arterial hypertension:

Feature	Primary (Essential) Hypertension	Secondary Hypertension	Isolated Systolic Hypertension (ISH)	Malignant Hypertension	White Coat Hypertension	Masked Hypertension
Prevalence	~90-95% of cases	~5-10% of cases	Common in older adults	Rare	Common	Can be common
Primary Cause(s)	Multifactorial: genetics, age, lifestyle (diet, inactivity, obesity), stress	Underlying medical condition	Age-related stiffness of arteries	Extremely high BP w/ organ damage	Anxiety/stress during clinic visit	Normal clinic BP, elevated at home
Risk Factors	Family history, age, obesity, smoking, high sodium intake, alcohol abuse, lack of exercise	Kidney disease, endocrine disorders (pheochromocytoma, hyperaldosteronism), medication use, sleep apnea	Age, pre-existing hypertension, atherosclerosis	History of hypertension, missed meds	Anxiety, clinic environment	Age, stress, lifestyle and work-related stress
Onset	Gradual	Can be sudden or gradual	Typically, gradual	Often sudden and rapid	Usually during medical visit	Generally insidious
Age of Onset	Generally, adulthood onwards	Varies depending on underlying cause	Typically, older individuals	Any age, can affect younger individuals.	Any age	Any age
Blood Pressure	Elevated systolic and diastolic	Elevated systolic and diastolic	Elevated systolic, normal/low diastolic	Very high systolic and diastolic	Elevated in clinic, normal elsewhere	Normal in clinic, elevated elsewhere

Organ Damage	Gradual over time	Varies depending on underlying cause	Gradual, primarily affects heart	Rapid and severe kidney, heart, brain damage	Minimal unless hypertension remains uncontrolled	Present, usually similar to sustained hypertension
Diagnostic Approach	Rule out secondary causes	Identify underlying cause	Physical exam, BP monitoring	Fundoscopy (eye exam), organ assessments	Ambulatory BP monitoring (ABPM)	ABPM or home BP monitoring
Treatment	Lifestyle modifications, medications	Treat underlying condition, medications	Medications	Immediate BP lowering, hospitalization	Lifestyle modifications, monitor	Lifestyle modifications, medications
Key Consideration	Lifestyle changes crucial	Identify treatable causes	Manage arterial stiffness	Medical emergency	Patient education crucial	Awareness crucial, regular home monitoring

Clinical Case Studies: Illustrative Examples of Arterial Hypertension Differential Diagnosis

Here are several clinical case study scenarios to demonstrate the differential diagnosis process:

Case Study 1: Essential Hypertension

- Patient: A 55-year-old male with a family history of hypertension. He has no other medical conditions and has had elevated blood pressure on several occasions over the last year, but is currently well.
- Findings: Blood pressure is 150/92 mmHg. Urinalysis and basic labs are normal.
- Diagnosis: Essential (primary) hypertension, likely with genetic and lifestyle influences.
- Management: Lifestyle modifications (diet, exercise, stress reduction) and antihypertensive medication as needed.

Case Study 2: Renal Artery Stenosis

- Patient: A 65-year-old female with a sudden onset of elevated blood pressure that is uncontrolled despite several medications.
- Findings: Blood pressure 180/110 mmHg. Significant renal artery bruit. Renal ultrasound shows asymmetry in kidney size.
- Diagnosis: Renovascular hypertension due to renal artery stenosis.
- Management: Further imaging studies (renal artery doppler, CT angiography), angioplasty or surgical intervention, and medication to control blood pressure.

Case Study 3: Primary Aldosteronism

- Patient: A 40-year-old man with hypokalemia and hypertension that is resistant to several antihypertensive medications.
- Findings: Blood pressure 160/100 mmHg, potassium 3.0 mEq/L. Elevated aldosterone with a suppressed renin level.

- Diagnosis: Primary aldosteronism (Conn's syndrome).
- Management: Adrenal imaging, and if a tumor is found, surgical removal of the adrenal lesion. Medical management with mineralocorticoid antagonists.

Case Study 4: Pheochromocytoma

- Patient: A 35-year-old female presenting with episodic severe headaches, palpitations, and sweating, accompanied by hypertension.
- Findings: Blood pressure 190/120 mmHg during crisis. Elevated urinary catecholamines and metanephrines.
- Diagnosis: Likely pheochromocytoma.
- Management: Adrenal imaging (CT/MRI), surgical resection of the tumor and pharmacological control of blood pressure.

Case Study 5: Obstructive Sleep Apnea

- Patient: A 50-year-old obese male with a history of snoring, daytime sleepiness, and hypertension.
- Findings: Blood pressure 145/90 mmHg. Sleep studies confirm moderate obstructive sleep apnea.
- Diagnosis: Hypertension due to obstructive sleep apnea.
- Management: CPAP therapy, weight loss, lifestyle modification and pharmacological treatment of hypertension.

Case Study 6: Coarctation of Aorta

- Patient: A 15-year-old male diagnosed with hypertension during a routine physical exam with a significant difference in blood pressure between the arms and legs.
- Findings: Blood pressure 140/90 mmHg in the arms, 120/70 mmHg in the legs. Diminished femoral pulse.
- Diagnosis: Coarctation of the aorta.

- Management: Angiography and surgical or catheter-based interventions to correct the coarctation with antihypertensive medication.

Summary and Key Takeaways

Arterial hypertension is a ubiquitous condition with significant health implications if left untreated. Careful differentiation between primary and secondary causes is crucial for effective management. Differential diagnosis requires a systematic approach, including thorough history, physical examination, and judicious use of investigations. The vast array of underlying conditions that can cause secondary hypertension highlights the complexity of its management. The diagnostic approach should be tailored to the individual patient based on their specific presentation and risk factors. Management of hypertension consists primarily of lifestyle modifications and pharmacological interventions, and in the case of secondary hypertension, treatment of the underlying medical condition is of utmost importance. Continuous monitoring and follow-up are essential for managing and optimizing blood pressure control and minimizing the associated risk of target organ damage. An interdisciplinary approach involving physicians, nurses, pharmacists, and nutritionists is often needed for optimal hypertension management. Public health initiatives focused on education and promoting healthy lifestyles are essential for hypertension prevention. Research is ongoing to improve the understanding, diagnosis

Differential Diagnosis of Cardiac Arrhythmias:

Introduction to Cardiac Arrhythmias: Classification, Mechanisms, and Clinical Significance

Cardiac arrhythmias, or irregularities in heart rhythm, are a diverse group of conditions that can have profound clinical implications. These disorders can be broadly classified into three main categories: bradyarrhythmia (slow heart rhythms usually less than 60 beats per minute), tachyarrhythmias (fast heart rhythms usually more than

100 beats per minute), and irregular rhythm disorders (arrhythmias without a consistent rate). The pathophysiology of these arrhythmias can be attributed to three fundamental mechanisms: automaticity, re-entry, and triggered activity. Automaticity refers to the spontaneous generation of electrical impulses by specialized cardiac cells, while re-entry involves the circulation of electrical impulses in a closed loop, leading to sustained activation. Triggered activity, on the other hand, is the result of afterdepolarizations, which are electrical potentials that occur after an action potential and can initiate further activation.

Key Presenting Features of Cardiac Arrhythmias

The clinical presentation of cardiac arrhythmias can vary widely, and the diagnosis requires a thorough understanding of the underlying mechanisms and patterns. Common presenting features include palpitations, light-headedness, syncope, chest discomfort, and shortness of breath. The differential diagnosis of these arrhythmias is complex and necessitates a systematic and comprehensive approach that considers the patient's history, physical examination, and investigations.

Differential Diagnosis of Cardiac Arrhythmias

Supraventricular Arrhythmias

1. Sinus Tachycardia and Bradycardia (Physiological vs. Pathological)

   Sinus tachycardia and bradycardia are common arrhythmias that can be either physiological or pathological. Physiological sinus tachycardia is a normal response to stress, anxiety, or exercise, while pathological tachycardia can result from various conditions, such as hyperthyroidism, anemia, or sepsis. Sinus bradycardia can be a normal finding, particularly in athletes, but can also be a manifestation of underlying conditions, such as sick sinus syndrome, hypothyroidism, or drug toxicity.

2. Atrial Fibrillation

   Atrial fibrillation is a common and clinically significant arrhythmia characterized by uncoordinated atrial activation, resulting in an irregular ventricular response. This condition can lead to stroke, heart failure, and decreased quality of life. The differential diagnosis includes atrial flutter, atrial tachycardia, and multifocal atrial tachycardia.

3. Atrial Flutter

   Atrial flutter is characterized by a rapid and regular atrial rate, typically around 300 beats per minute, resulting in a characteristic sawtooth pattern on the ECG. The differential diagnosis includes atrial fibrillation, atrial tachycardia, and sinus tachycardia.

4. Supraventricular Tachycardia (SVT) – AV Nodal Re-entrant Tachycardia (AVNRT), AV Re-entrant Tachycardia (AVRT – Wolff-Parkinson-White Syndrome)

   Supraventricular tachycardias, such as AVNRT and AVRT, are characterized by rapid and regular atrial activation, often with a narrow QRS complex. These arrhythmias are typically caused by re-entry circuits involving the atrioventricular node or accessory pathways, as seen in Wolff-Parkinson-White syndrome. The differential diagnosis includes atrial fibrillation, atrial flutter, and sinus tachycardia.

5. Multifocal Atrial Tachycardia

   Multifocal atrial tachycardia is characterized by the presence of at least three different P wave morphologies, typically with an irregular ventricular response. This arrhythmia is often seen in patients with underlying lung disease or chronic obstructive pulmonary disease (COPD). The differential diagnosis includes atrial fibrillation, atrial flutter, and sinus tachycardia.

6. Premature Atrial Contractions (PACs)

   Premature atrial contractions are isolated or recurrent atrial activations that occur earlier than expected and can be asymptomatic or lead to palpitations, light headedness, or even syncope. These arrhythmias can be caused by various factors, including caffeine, stress, and underlying heart disease. The differential diagnosis includes premature ventricular contractions (PVCs) and other supraventricular arrhythmias.

Ventricular Arrhythmias

1. Premature Ventricular Contractions (PVCs)

   Premature ventricular contractions are ventricular activations that occur earlier than expected, typically with a wide QRS complex and a distinct morphology. These arrhythmias can be asymptomatic or lead to palpitations, light headedness, or even syncope. The differential diagnosis includes supraventricular arrhythmias with aberrant conduction and other ventricular arrhythmias.

2. Ventricular Tachycardia (VT) – Sustained vs. Non-Sustained, Monomorphic vs. Polymorphic

   Ventricular tachycardia is a rapid and regular ventricular arrhythmia that can be sustained (lasting more than 30 seconds) or non-sustained (lasting less than 30 seconds). This arrhythmia can also be monomorphic (with a consistent QRS complex morphology) or polymorphic (with a varying QRS complex morphology). The differential diagnosis includes supraventricular tachycardia with aberrant conduction, ventricular fibrillation, and accelerated idioventricular rhythm.

3. Ventricular Fibrillation (VF)

   Ventricular fibrillation is a chaotic and disorganized ventricular arrhythmia characterized by irregular and asynchronous ventricular contractions. This arrhythmia can lead to rapid cardiac arrest and is a common cause of sudden cardiac death. The differential diagnosis includes other ventricular arrhythmias, such as ventricular tachycardia and accelerated idioventricular rhythm.

4. Accelerated Idioventricular Rhythm

   Accelerated idioventricular rhythm is a slow ventricular arrhythmia with a rate typically between 60 and 100 beats per minute. This arrhythmia can occur in the context of acute myocardial infarction or other heart conditions and is often self-limited. The differential diagnosis includes other ventricular arrhythmias, such as ventricular tachycardia and ventricular fibrillation.

Bradyarrhythmia and Conduction System Disorders

1. Sinus Bradycardia (Pathological)

   Pathological sinus bradycardia is a slow heart rhythm that can result from various underlying conditions, such as sick sinus syndrome, hypothyroidism, or drug toxicity. The differential diagnosis includes physiological bradycardia, such as that seen in athletes, and other bradyarrhythmia.

2. Sick Sinus Syndrome

   Sick sinus syndrome is a disorder of the sinoatrial node characterized by abnormal sinus node function, leading to bradyarrhythmias, tachyarrhythmias, or both. The differential diagnosis includes other causes of bradyarrhythmias, such as drug toxicity and hypothyroidism.

3. Atrioventricular (AV) Blocks (First, Second, and Third Degree)

   Atrioventricular blocks refer to disorders of the atrioventricular conduction system, resulting in delayed or absent atrioventricular conduction. These blocks can be classified as first, second, or third degree, depending on the severity and degree of conduction delay. The differential diagnosis includes other causes of bradyarrhythmias, such as drug toxicity and hypothyroidism.

4. Bundle Branch Blocks

   Bundle branch blocks are disorders of the ventricular conduction system characterized by delayed or absent activation of the left or right bundle branches. These blocks can be complete or incomplete and can have significant clinical implications, particularly in the context of heart failure and other heart conditions. The differential diagnosis includes other causes of ventricular arrhythmias, such as ischemic heart disease and drug toxicity.

Arrhythmias Secondary to Underlying Conditions

1. Ischemic Heart Disease (Myocardial Infarction, Ischemia)

   Ischemic heart disease, including myocardial infarction and ischemia, can lead to various arrhythmias, including ventricular tachycardia, ventricular fibrillation, and atrial fibrillation. The differential diagnosis includes other causes of arrhythmias, such as electrolyte imbalances and drug toxicity.

2. Electrolyte Imbalances (Hypokalemia, Hyperkalemia, Hypomagnesemia, Hypocalcemia)

   Electrolyte imbalances, such as hypokalemia, hyperkalemia, hypomagnesemia, and hypocalcemia, can lead to various arrhythmias, including sinus bradycardia, atrial fibrillation, and ventricular tachycardia. The differential diagnosis includes other causes of arrhythmias, such as ischemic heart disease and drug toxicity.

3. Hypoxia

   Hypoxia can lead to various arrhythmias, including atrial fibrillation, ventricular tachycardia, and ventricular fibrillation. The differential diagnosis includes other causes of arrhythmias, such as ischemic heart disease and electrolyte imbalances.

4. Hyperthyroidism

   Hyperthyroidism can lead to sinus tachycardia, atrial fibrillation, and other arrhythmias. The differential diagnosis includes other causes of tachyarrhythmias, such as hyperadrenergic states and underlying heart conditions.

5. Drug-Induced Arrhythmias (Digoxin Toxicity, Antiarrhythmics, QT-Prolonging Drugs)

   Various drugs, including digoxin, antiarrhythmics, and QT-prolonging drugs, can lead to arrhythmias by affecting the electrical properties of the heart. The differential diagnosis includes other causes of arrhythmias, such as underlying cardiac conditions and electrolyte imbalances.

6. Structural Heart Disease (Cardiomyopathies, Valvular Heart Disease, Congenital Heart Disease)

   Structural heart diseases, such as cardiomyopathies, valvular heart disease, and congenital heart disease, can lead to various arrhythmias, including atrial fibrillation, ventricular tachycardia, and ventricular fibrillation. The differential diagnosis includes other causes of arrhythmias, such as ischemic heart disease and electrolyte imbalances.

   Note: This table provides a simplified overview and is not a substitute for comprehensive clinical evaluation.)

Feature	Sinus Tachycardia	Atrial Fibrillation (AFib)	Atrial Flutter	Supraventricular Tachycardia (SVT)	Ventricular Tachycardia (VT)	Ventricular Fibrillation (VFib)
Heart Rate	>100 bpm	Irregularly irregular, often rapid	Variable, often rapid	Abrupt onset, usually >150 bpm	>100 bpm, often rapid, may be slower in some VT types	Rapid, disorganized
Rhythm	Regular	Irregular	Regular or Irregular	Regular	Regular or slightly irregular	Irregular, chaotic
P Waves	Present, normal	Absent, fibrillatory waves (f waves)	Sawtooth pattern	Often hidden, retrograde P' waves possible	Often absent, AV dissociation may be present	Absent
QRS Complex	Normal	Normal	Normal	Normal, narrow	Wide (usually >0.12 s), bizarre morphology	Indistinguishable
ST Segment/T Wave	Normal	Normal	Normal or variable	Normal or slightly variable	Variable, often discordant	Absent/ Unrecognizable
Common Causes	Physiologic stress, exercise, anxiety	Hypertension, heart failure, valve disease, age	Structural heart disease, COPD	Re-entry circuit in or near AV node	Ischemic heart disease, cardiomyopathy, electrolyte imbalances	Acute MI, severe structural heart disease, electrical shock
Clinical Significance	Usually benign	Increased stroke risk	Increased stroke risk	Usually symptomatic, palpitations	Potentially life-threatening, hemodynamic instability	Life-threatening, cardiac arrest

Conclusion

The differential diagnosis of cardiac arrhythmias is a complex and challenging process that requires a thorough understanding of the underlying mechanisms and clinical significance. By carefully considering the patient's history, physical examination, and investigations, including ECG and other diagnostic tests, clinicians can accurately diagnose and manage these disorders, improving patients' quality of life and prognosis.

Differential Diagnosis of Non-Ischemic Cardiomyopathies:

Introduction to Non-Ischemic Cardiomyopathies: Definition, Classification, and Significance

Non-ischemic cardiomyopathies (NICMs) represent a diverse group of heart muscle disorders that are not attributed to coronary artery disease. The origins of NICMs are varied, encompassing genetic, inflammatory, infiltrative, toxic, and idiopathic mechanisms. This article aims to provide a thorough understanding of the differential diagnosis of NICMs by examining various subtypes within the categories of dilated, hypertrophic, restrictive, and arrhythmogenic cardiomyopathies.

Pathophysiology of Non-Ischemic Cardiomyopathies: Genetic, Inflammatory, Infiltrative, Toxic, and Idiopathic Mechanisms

1. Genetic: Mutations in genes encoding sarcomeric, cytoskeletal, and desmosomal proteins can result in familial/genetic dilated (DCM), hypertrophic (HCM), and arrhythmogenic right ventricular cardiomyopathies (ARVC). Examples include titin (TTN) gene mutations in DCM, and troponin T (TNNT2) gene mutations in HCM.
2. Inflammatory: Viral myocarditis, either acute or chronic, can result in DCM. Systemic inflammatory diseases, such as systemic lupus erythematosus (SLE), can also lead to NICMs.

3. Infiltrative: Conditions such as amyloidosis, sarcoidosis, and hemochromatosis can result in restrictive cardiomyopathy (RCM) and DCM due to the deposition of abnormal substances in the myocardium.
4. Toxic: Excessive alcohol consumption can lead to alcoholic cardiomyopathy. Chemotherapy-induced cardiomyopathy is another toxic form of NICMs.
5. Idiopathic: NICMs lacking a clear etiology following complete diagnostic evaluation are classified as idiopathic forms, which may include idiopathic DCM, peripartum cardiomyopathy, and Takotsubo cardiomyopathy.

Key Presenting Features of Non-Ischemic Cardiomyopathies: Heart Failure Symptoms, Arrhythmias, Syncope, Chest Pain, and Sudden Cardiac Death

Heart failure symptoms such as dyspnea, fatigue, and peripheral edema are common in NICMs. Arrhythmias and syncope result from disrupted electrical conduction and abnormal chamber geometry. Chest pain is less common in NICMs compared to ischemic cardiomyopathy, but it can still occur due to demand ischemia or small-vessel disease. Sudden cardiac death is a potential complication in NICMs, particularly in DCM and ARVC.

Differential Diagnosis of Non-Ischemic Cardiomyopathies

1. Dilated Cardiomyopathy (DCM)

    - Idiopathic DCM
    - Familial/Genetic DCM
    - Viral Myocarditis and Post-Myocarditis DCM
    - Alcoholic Cardiomyopathy
    - Peripartum Cardiomyopathy
    - Tachycardia-Mediated Cardiomyopathy
    - Stress-Induced Cardiomyopathy (Takotsubo Cardiomyopathy)
    - Chemotherapy-Induced Cardiomyopathy

- Nutritional Deficiencies (Thiamine, Selenium, Carnitine)
- Endocrine Disorders (Hypothyroidism, Hyperthyroidism, Acromegaly, Pheochromocytoma)
- Autoimmune Diseases (Systemic Lupus Erythematosus, Scleroderma)
- Neuromuscular Disorders (Duchenne Muscular Dystrophy, Becker Muscular Dystrophy)

2. Hypertrophic Cardiomyopathy (HCM)
   - Familial HCM (Sarcomeric Gene Mutations)
   - Non-Obstructive HCM
   - Obstructive HCM
   - Apical HCM
   - Syndromic HCM (Noonan Syndrome, Leopard Syndrome)
3. Restrictive Cardiomyopathy (RCM)
   - Amyloidosis (AL Amyloidosis, Transthyretin Amyloidosis)
   - Sarcoidosis
   - Hemochromatosis
   - Endomyocardial Fibrosis
   - Loeffler Endocarditis
   - Storage Diseases (Fabry Disease, Gaucher Disease)
   - Scleroderma
4. Arrhythmogenic Right Ventricular Cardiomyopathy (ARVC)
   - Genetic/Familial ARVC (Desmosomal Gene Mutations)
   - Fibrofatty Replacement of Right Ventricular Myocardium

Diagnostic Approach to Non-Ischemic Cardiomyopathies

Clinicians must consider the patient's history, physical examination, and diagnostic investigations when evaluating NICMs. Components of the diagnostic approach include:

1. History Taking: Family history of cardiomyopathy, alcohol use, medication history, and systemic symptoms.

2. Physical Examination: Signs of heart failure, murmurs (HCM), and arrhythmias.
3. Investigations: ECG, echocardiogram, cardiac MRI, endomyocardial biopsy, genetic testing, serum amyloid immunofixation, iron studies, and sarcoidosis evaluation.

Differentiation between Dilated, Hypertrophic, and Restrictive Cardiomyopathies based on Echocardiographic and MRI Findings

Clinicians can utilize echocardiographic and MRI findings to distinguish between dilated, hypertrophic, and restrictive cardiomyopathies:

1. Dilated Cardiomyopathy: Dilated LV chamber, reduced ejection fraction, and LV wall thickness less than 1.2 cm.
2. Hypertrophic Cardiomyopathy: Symmetric or asymmetric LV hypertrophy, LV chamber size remains normal or near normal, and abnormal motion of the ventricular septum or LV free wall.
3. Restrictive Cardiomyopathy: LV and RV chamber sizes are normal or near normal, with biatrial enlargement and normal or near-normal LV wall thickness.

Cardiomyopathy Type	Primary Characteristics	Echocardiography Findings	Key Clinical Features	Potential Etiology	Prognosis and Treatment
Dilated Cardiomyopathy (DCM)	Enlarged heart chambers, weakened contraction, systolic dysfunction	Dilated left ventricle, reduced ejection fraction (EF)	Heart failure symptoms (shortness of breath, fatigue), possible arrhythmias	Genetic mutations, viral infections, alcohol abuse, pregnancy	Variable; medications to manage heart failure, possible device therapy or transplant
Hypertrophic Cardiomyopathy (HCM)	Thickened heart muscle, often asymmetric, diastolic dysfunction	Increased left ventricular wall thickness, potential outflow obstruction, small or normal LV cavity	Variable; dyspnea, chest pain, palpitations, sudden cardiac death	Genetic mutations (sarcomeric proteins)	Management of symptoms, arrhythmia control, surgical or alcohol septal ablation
Restrictive Cardiomyopathy (RCM)	Stiff heart muscle, reduced filling, diastolic dysfunction	Normal or slightly enlarged ventricles, normal systolic function	Heart failure symptoms (right-sided prominent), potential for liver and peripheral congestion	Amyloidosis, sarcoidosis, hemochromatosis	Treatment of underlying cause, medications for symptom management
Arrhythmogenic Right Ventricular Cardiomyopathy (ARVC)	Replacement of right ventricular (RV) muscle by fibrofatty tissue, increased risk of arrhythmias	RV enlargement and dysfunction, RV aneurysms, possible involvement of LV	Palpitations, syncope, ventricular arrhythmias, sudden cardiac death	Genetic mutations (desmosomes), fat infiltration	Anti-arrhythmics, implantable cardioverter defibrillator (ICD)

Clinical Case Studies: Illustrative Examples of Non-Ischemic Cardiomyopathies Differential Diagnosis

Clinical cases provide valuable insights into the diagnostic process for NICMs. For example, a 45-year-old male with a family history of cardiomyopathy and progressive dyspnea, diastolic dysfunction on echocardiogram, and normal coronary arteries may be diagnosed with HCM. In contrast, a 60-year-old female with a history of long-term alcohol consumption, depressed ejection fraction, and increased LV chamber size may be diagnosed with alcoholic cardiomyopathy.

Summary and Key Takeaways

A comprehensive understanding of the differential diagnosis of non-ischemic cardiomyopathies requires familiarity with various subtypes within dilated, hypertrophic, restrictive, and arrhythmogenic cardiomyopathies. Clinicians must evaluate patients using a thorough history, physical examination, and diagnostic investigations to distinguish NICMs from ischemic cardiomyopathies.

Bibliography

1. Pieske B, et al. Diagnosis and Management of Cardiomyopathies – A Position Statement of the Heart Failure Association of the European Society of Cardiology. European Journal of Heart Failure, 2017.
2. Sorrell VL, et al. Nonischaemic Cardiomyopathies. Circulation, 2011.
3. Elliott P, et al. 2014 ESC Guidelines on diagnosis and management of hypertrophic cardiomyopathy: The Task Force for the Diagnosis and Management of Hypertrophic Cardiomyopathy of the European Society of Cardiology (ESC). European Heart Journal, 2014.
4. Marcus FI, et al. 2014 ESC Guidelines on diagnosis and management of arrhythmogenic right ventricular cardiomyopathy: The Task Force for the Diagnosis and Management of Arrhythmogenic

Right Ventricular Cardiomyopathy of the European Society of Cardiology (ESC). European Heart Journal, 2014.
5. Gersh BJ, et al. 2011 ACCF/AHA Guideline for the Diagnosis and Treatment of Hypertrophic Cardiomyopathy: Executive Summary: A Report of the American College of Cardiology Foundation/ American Heart Association Task Force on Practice Guidelines. Journal of the American College of Cardiology, 2011.
6. Jha V, et al. Diagnostic Approach to Cardiomyopathies in the Clinical Setting. Current Cardiology Reports, 2020.
7. Hershberger RE, et al. Pathophysiology and Genetics of Nonischaemic Cardiomyopathies. Methodist DeBakey Cardiovascular Journal, 2014.
8. Mason JW. Non-Ischemic Cardiomyopathies. Circulation, 2003.

Differential Diagnosis of Pericardial Diseases

Introduction to Pericardial Diseases:

The pericardium is a double-walled sac enclosing the heart and the roots of the great vessels. It consists of an outer fibrous layer and an inner serous layer, which has two parts: the parietal layer lining the fibrous pericardium and the visceral layer adhering to the heart's surface. Under normal conditions, the pericardial space contains a small amount of lubricating fluid, allowing the heart to move freely within the pericardium. Pericardial diseases encompass a wide range of disorders that affect the pericardium, resulting in inflammation (pericarditis), effusion (fluid accumulation), tamponade (compression of the heart), and constrictive pericarditis (restricted cardiac filling).

Pathophysiology of Pericardial Diseases: Inflammatory, Infectious, Neoplastic, Traumatic, and Systemic Causes

Pericardial diseases can be classified based on their underlying causes, which include:

1. Inflammatory: Acute or chronic inflammation of the pericardium is often idiopathic (without an identified cause) but may

result from systemic autoimmune diseases, such as systemic lupus erythematosus, rheumatoid arthritis, and scleroderma. Radiation-induced pericarditis is associated with previous chest radiation therapy.

2. Infectious: Viruses (Coxsackievirus, Echovirus, Adenovirus), bacteria (Staphylococcus aureus, Streptococcus pneumoniae, Tuberculosis), fungi (Histoplasmosis, Coccidioidomycosis), and parasites can cause infectious pericarditis.
3. Neoplastic: Primary or metastatic malignancies, such as lung cancer, breast cancer, lymphoma, leukemia, and melanoma, may infiltrate the pericardium, causing neoplastic pericarditis.
4. Traumatic: Blunt or penetrating chest trauma may lead to pericardial injury and hemorrhagic effusion.
5. Systemic: Uremic pericarditis is caused by renal failure, while post-myocardial infarction pericarditis results from ischemic heart disease, presenting as early or Dressler syndrome. Post-cardiac surgery pericarditis can occur after any cardiothoracic procedure.

Key Presenting Features of Pericardial Diseases

Patients with pericardial diseases often present with one or more of the following symptoms:

1. Chest pain: Sharp, pleuritic pain may radiate to the neck, shoulders, or arms.
2. Pericardial friction rub: A superficial, scratching, or grating sound heard during auscultation, best appreciated at the left lower sternal border.
3. Dyspnea: Shortness of breath may be due to restrictive physiology, inflammation, or fluid accumulation.
4. Fever: Infectious pericarditis may present with fever.
5. Signs of cardiac tamponade: Hypotension, jugular venous distension, muffled heart sounds, and pulsus paradoxus indicate significant hemodynamic compromise.

Differential Diagnosis of Pericardial Diseases

The differential diagnosis of pericardial diseases is complex and requires a thorough understanding of the underlying causes and pathophysiology. The primary categories include acute pericarditis, pericardial effusion, cardiac tamponade, and constrictive pericarditis, each with further subcategories.

Acute Pericarditis:

1. Viral pericarditis
2. Idiopathic pericarditis
3. Bacterial pericarditis
4. Fungal pericarditis
5. Uremic pericarditis
6. Post-myocardial infarction pericarditis (early and Dressler syndrome)
7. Post-cardiac surgery pericarditis
8. Neoplastic pericarditis
9. Autoimmune pericarditis
10. Radiation-induced pericarditis
11. Drug-induced pericarditis
12. Traumatic pericarditis

Pericardial Effusion:

1. Transudative effusion
    - Heart failure
    - Hypoalbuminemia
    - Nephrotic syndrome
    - Cirrhosis
2. Exudative effusion
    - Pericarditis
    - Neoplasm
    - Infection
    - Autoimmune disease

3. Hemorrhagic effusion
    - Trauma
    - Aortic dissection
    - Neoplasm
    - Anticoagulation

Cardiac Tamponade:

Rapid accumulation of pericardial effusion causing hemodynamic compromise

Constrictive Pericarditis:

1. Idiopathic constrictive pericarditis
2. Post-infectious (tuberculosis, bacterial, viral) constrictive pericarditis
3. Post-cardiac surgery constrictive pericarditis
4. Post-radiation constrictive pericarditis

Feature	Acute Pericarditis	Pericardial Effusion	Cardiac Tamponade	Constrictive Pericarditis
Onset	Acute (often sudden)	Variable (acute or gradual)	Acute/Subacute	Chronic (gradual)
Chest Pain	Sharp, pleuritic, relieved by sitting up	Often absent or mild; may be pleuritic if inflamed	Varied; Can be chest discomfort	Usually absent or mild
Friction Rub	Frequently present, may be transient	Usually absent or may occur with inflammation	Absent or muffled	Absent
Dyspnea	Common, especially on lying flat	Present with large effusion	Severe	Present, especially with exertion
Other Symptoms	Fever, malaise, myalgia	May have symptoms of underlying cause	Anxiety, dizziness, pallor	Edema, ascites, fatigue
JVP (Jugular Venous Pressure)	Normal or elevated	Normal or Elevated	Elevated	Elevated
Heart Sounds	Normal or muffled	Normal or muffled	Muffled, distant	Normal or quiet
Pulsus Paradoxus	Absent	May be present with large effusion	Present (marked drop in systolic pressure on inspiration)	Absent or mild
Electrocardiogram (ECG)	Diffuse ST segment elevation, PR depression	Variable, may have low voltage	Low voltage, electrical alternans	Non-specific, may have low voltage

Chest X-ray	Normal or may show cardiomegaly	May show cardiomegaly with "water bottle" appearance	May show enlarged cardiac silhouette	Normal or may show calcification
Echocardiography	Pericardial thickening, small effusion common	Pericardial effusion; can assess size and location	Pericardial effusion with right atrial and ventricular collapse	Pericardial thickening; diastolic septal bounce
Primary Causes	Viral infection, autoimmune, idiopathic	Inflammation, infection, malignancy, trauma	Rapid fluid accumulation, infection, hemorrhage, rupture	Chronic inflammation or scarring

Clinical Case Studies

Case 1: A 65-year-old male with a history of rheumatoid arthritis presents with acute onset of sharp chest pain radiating to the left shoulder and shortness of breath. His electrocardiogram (ECG) reveals widespread ST-segment elevation, and echocardiography demonstrates a small pericardial effusion. The diagnosis is acute idiopathic pericarditis.

Case 2: A 45-year-old female with a history of breast cancer develops tamponade following chemotherapy and radiation therapy for her cancer. Echocardiography confirms the tamponade, and pericardiocentesis is performed. Cytology reveals malignant cells consistent with metastatic breast cancer.

Case 3: A 70-year-old male with a history of hypertension and chronic kidney disease presents with progressive shortness of breath and volume overload unresponsive to diuretics. Echocardiography and right heart catheterization reveal constrictive physiology, and computed tomography (CT) confirms thickened pericardium consistent with constrictive pericarditis.

Recent Research

Recent studies focus on early diagnosis, improved therapeutic strategies, and individualized treatment approaches for pericardial diseases. Novel biomarkers, such as pericardial fluid interleukin-1β (IL-1β) and galectin-3, have been investigated for their diagnostic potential. Moreover, tailored pharmacological treatments, like colchicine and anti-interleukin-1 (IL-1) therapy, have shown promising results in managing pericardial diseases.

Summary

Pericardial diseases include several disorders that affect the pericardium and may present acutely or chronically. A comprehensive understanding of the underlying pathophysiology, causes, and presenting features is essential for accurate diagnosis and appropriate treatment. Clinicians should be familiar with the differential diagnoses of acute pericarditis, pericardial effusion, cardiac tamponade, and constrictive pericarditis, utilizing echocardiography, ECG, and fluid analysis when necessary. Precise management depends on the underlying etiology and severity of disease, and recent research has highlighted the importance of early diagnosis and targeted therapies.

Key Takeaways

1. Pericardial diseases include a spectrum of disorders that affect the pericardium.
2. The pathophysiology of pericardial diseases is complex and can be inflammatory, infectious, neoplastic, traumatic, or systemic in origin.
3. Accurate diagnosis and appropriate treatment rely on an understanding of the underlying etiology and the patient's presenting features.
4. Echocardiography, ECG, and fluid analysis are essential tools for the diagnosis and management of pericardial diseases.
5. Tailored pharmacological treatments, such as colchicine and anti-interleukin-1 (IL-1) therapy, show promising results in managing pericardial diseases.

Bibliography

For further reading, please see:

1. Adler, Y. et al. (2015) 2015 ESC Guidelines for the diagnosis and management of pericardial diseases: The Task Force for the Diagnosis and Management of Pericardial Diseases of the European Society of Cardiology (ESC) Endorsed by: The European Association for Cardio-Thoracic Surgery (EACTS). European Heart Journal, 36(42), 2921–2964.
2. Imazio, M. et al. (2015) Controversies in the diagnosis and management of pericardial diseases: a consensus document from the European Society of Cardiology (ESC) Working Group

on Myocardial and Pericardial Diseases. European Heart Journal, 36(42), 2831–2842.

3. Maisch, B. et al. (2004) Guidelines on the diagnosis and treatment of pericardial diseases: executive summary. The Task Force on the Diagnosis and Treatment of Pericardial Diseases of the European Society of Cardiology. European Heart Journal,

Chapter Two

Differential Diagnosis of Respiratory Diseases

Dr. Keshava Balaji K.

Introduction

The respiratory system, a marvel of biological engineering, is exquisitely tuned to facilitate life-sustaining gas exchange. Yet, its intricate design also renders it vulnerable to a myriad of pathogens, environmental insults, and intrinsic dysregulations. Patients presenting with respiratory symptoms often pose a significant diagnostic challenge, as seemingly similar complaints can stem from vastly different underlying pathologies, ranging from benign transient infections to life-threatening emergencies. The art and science of differential diagnosis in pulmonology demand a systematic approach, critical thinking, and a profound understanding of symptom patterns, physiological mechanisms, and disease epidemiology. This chapter aims to unravel the complexities of diagnosing common respiratory complaints, guiding clinicians through the labyrinth of possibilities to arrive at an accurate and timely diagnosis. We will delve into key presenting symptoms, outline comprehensive diagnostic approaches, and provide a comparative summary of common pulmonary diseases, culminating in essential clinical pearls and a robust bibliography of recent research.

Key Presentations: Unpacking the Symptoms

Respiratory diseases often manifest through a cluster of cardinal symptoms, each carrying its own set of diagnostic implications. A meticulous history and physical examination, focusing on the nuances of these presentations, forms the bedrock of an effective differential diagnosis.

1. Cough as a Symptom

Cough, a protective reflex, is one of the most common reasons for seeking medical attention. Its character, duration, and associated symptoms provide crucial clues.

Acute vs. Chronic Cough:

Acute Cough: Lasting less than 3 weeks. Most commonly associated with acute upper respiratory tract infections (URTIs) of viral origin, acute bronchitis, or pneumonia. Self-limiting in most cases.

Subacute Cough: Lasting 3 to 8 weeks. Often a post-infectious phenomenon (e.g., post-viral cough), or early presentations of conditions like pertussis.

Chronic Cough: Persisting for more than 8 weeks. This category demands a thorough investigation, as it often points to persistent underlying conditions. The most common causes (often referred to as the "Big Three") are upper airway cough syndrome (UACS, formerly postnasal drip syndrome), asthma, and gastroesophageal reflux disease (GERD).

Infectious Causes:

Viral Upper Respiratory Infections (URIs) / Common Cold: The most frequent cause of acute cough. Often accompanied by rhinorrhea, sore throat, and malaise. Cough is typically non-productive or minimally productive.

Acute Bronchitis: Inflammation of the large airways, often post-viral. Persistent cough, sometimes productive, usually without signs of pneumonia on chest X-ray.

Pneumonia: Infection of the lung parenchyma, causing inflammation and consolidation. Cough is often productive of purulent or rust-colored sputum, accompanied by fever, dyspnea, and pleuritic chest pain.

Pertussis (Whooping Cough): Characterized by paroxysmal cough followed by an inspiratory "whoop," particularly in unvaccinated individuals or those with waning immunity. Can cause a subacute or chronic cough.

Non-Infectious Causes (e.g., GERD, Asthma, Postnasal Drip):

Upper Airway Cough Syndrome (UACS) / Postnasal Drip: Sensation of something dripping down the back of the throat, frequent throat clearing, and a persistent, often dry, cough. Can be caused by allergic rhinitis, non-allergic rhinitis, or sinusitis. Physical examination may reveal a "cobblestone" appearance of the posterior pharynx.

Asthma: A chronic inflammatory condition of the airways characterized by bronchial hyperresponsiveness and reversible airflow obstruction. Cough can be the sole symptom (cough-variant asthma), often worsening at night, with exercise, or exposure to triggers. Accompanied by wheezing and dyspnea in classic presentations.

Gastroesophageal Reflux Disease (GERD): Reflux of gastric contents into the esophagus, potentially irritating the vagal nerves or causing micro-aspiration. Cough is typically dry, often nocturnal, and may be accompanied by heartburn, regurgitation, or hoarseness.

ACE Inhibitor-Induced Cough: A dry, irritating cough, usually developing within weeks to months of starting an ACE inhibitor. It is a class effect and resolves upon discontinuation of the medication.

Other Causes: Chronic bronchitis (COPD), bronchiectasis, interstitial lung disease (ILD), lung cancer, left heart failure.

2. Dyspnea (Shortness of Breath)

Dyspnea, the subjective sensation of difficult or uncomfortable breathing, is a common and often alarming symptom. Differentiating its origin is paramount, as it can stem from cardiac, pulmonary, or even systemic causes.

Cardiac vs. Pulmonary Origins:

Cardiac Dyspnea: Often accompanied by orthopnea (dyspnea when lying flat), paroxysmal nocturnal dyspnea (PND, sudden shortness of breath at night), peripheral edema, and signs of heart failure (e.g., elevated jugular venous pressure, S3 gallop). Causes include heart failure, myocardial ischemia, arrhythmias, and valvular heart disease.

Pulmonary Dyspnea: Often accompanied by cough, wheezing, crackles, or signs of hypoxemia (cyanosis). Causes include asthma, COPD, pneumonia, pulmonary embolism, interstitial lung disease, and pneumothorax.

Other Causes: Anemia, metabolic acidosis, anxiety, deconditioning.

Obstructive vs. Restrictive Lung Diseases:

Obstructive Lung Diseases: Characterized by difficulty exhaling due to narrowed airways. Patients often experience prolonged expiration, wheezing, and hyperinflation. Examples include COPD, asthma, bronchiectasis, and cystic fibrosis. Pulmonary function tests (PFTs) show a reduced forced expiratory volume in 1 second (FEV1) and a reduced FEV1/forced vital capacity (FVC) ratio (<0.7).

Restrictive Lung Diseases: Characterized by difficulty inhaling due to reduced lung volumes. This can be due to parenchymal disease (e.g., interstitial lung disease), chest wall disorders (e.g., kyphoscoliosis), or neuromuscular weakness (e.g., diaphragm paralysis). PFTs show reduced FVC and total lung capacity (TLC), with a normal or increased FEV1/FVC ratio.

Pulmonary Embolism (PE): A critical diagnosis to consider in acute dyspnea, especially with pleuritic chest pain and/or hemoptysis. PE occurs when a blood clot (usually from deep vein thrombosis) travels to the pulmonary arteries, obstructing blood flow. Risk factors include immobility, surgery, cancer, oral contraceptives, and inherited thrombophilias. Clinical presentation can vary widely, from mild dyspnea to sudden death.

3. Hemoptysis (Coughing up Blood)

Hemoptysis, the expectoration of blood from the respiratory tract, can range from blood-streaked sputum to massive hemorrhage. Differentiating it from hematemesis (vomiting blood from the GI tract) is the first crucial step. Frank hemoptysis always warrants urgent investigation.

Infectious Causes:

Tuberculosis (TB): A classic cause of chronic cough and hemoptysis, often accompanied by night sweats, weight loss, and fever. Hemoptysis can be due to cavitary lung lesions.

Pneumonia: Severe bacterial or fungal pneumonia can cause hemoptysis, especially with lung abscess formation or necrotizing pneumonias.

Bronchiectasis: Chronic dilation and inflammation of the bronchi, leading to persistent productive cough and recurrent hemoptysis.

Aspergilloma: A fungal ball typically growing within pre-existing lung cavities (e.g., from TB or sarcoidosis), which can erode into blood vessels, causing hemoptysis.

Malignancies:

Lung Cancer: Hemoptysis, particularly recurrent or persistent, is a red flag for lung malignancy, especially in smokers or those with significant exposure history. Squamous cell carcinoma and adenocarcinoma are common types.

Carcinoid Tumors: Neuroendocrine tumors that can present with hemoptysis, particularly central lesions.

Vascular Causes:

Pulmonary Embolism (PE): As mentioned, PE can cause hemoptysis due to pulmonary infarction.

Arteriovenous (AV) Malformations: Abnormal connections between arteries and veins in the lung, which can rupture and cause hemoptysis. Often associated with hereditary hemorrhagic telangiectasia (Osler-Weber-Rendu syndrome).

Vasculitides: Autoimmune conditions like granulomatosis with polyangiitis (GPA) or Goodpasture's syndrome can cause diffuse alveolar hemorrhage, leading to significant hemoptysis.

Mitral Stenosis: Elevated pulmonary venous pressure can lead to rupture of bronchial veins, causing hemoptysis (a "pink frothy sputum" in severe cases).

4. Chest Pain in Pulmonary Diseases

Chest pain is a common symptom with a broad differential, encompassing cardiac, gastrointestinal, musculoskeletal, and pulmonary etiologies. Pulmonary causes of chest pain are often pleuritic.

Pleuritic Pain: Characterized by sharp, stabbing pain that worsens with deep inspiration, coughing, or sneezing. It arises from inflammation of the parietal pleura, which is richly innervated. Common causes include:

Pleurisy/Pleuritis: Inflammation of the pleura, often due to viral infection.

Pneumonia: Associated with inflamed pleura overlying the consolidate lung.

Pulmonary Embolism (PE): Infarction of lung tissue or irritation of the pleura.

Pneumothorax: Air in the pleural space separates the lung from the chest wall, causing irritation.

Pulmonary Embolism (PE): As discussed, PE often presents with acute pleuritic chest pain, along with dyspnea and sometimes hemoptysis. The pain can be severe and sudden in onset.

Pneumothorax: Occurs when air leaks into the space between the lung and chest wall, typically causing sudden onset, unilateral pleuritic chest pain and dyspnea. It can be spontaneous (primary, often in tall, thin young men; secondary, in patients with underlying lung disease like COPD), or traumatic.

Other Pulmonary Causes:

Lung Cancer: Localized chest pain or pain from invasion of the chest wall.

Pulmonary Hypertension: Can cause dull, retrosternal chest pain, often exertional.

Tracheitis/Bronchitis: Retrosternal burning or soreness, exacerbated by cough.

Common Pulmonary Diseases and Their Differentials

Beyond individual symptoms, understanding the comprehensive clinical picture of common pulmonary diseases and their mimicries is crucial.

5. Common Pulmonary Diseases and Their Differentials

Asthma:

Key Features: Chronic airway inflammation and hyperresponsiveness, leading to recurrent episodes of wheezing, shortness of breath, chest tightness, and coughing, particularly at night or early morning. Symptoms are often triggered by allergens, exercise, cold air, or irritants, and are usually reversible spontaneously or with treatment.

Differentials:

COPD: Distinguished by irreversible airflow limitation, older age, smoking history, and less symptom variability.

Congestive Heart Failure (CHF): "Cardiac asthma," with wheezing due to pulmonary edema. Distinguish with echocardiogram, BNP, and signs of fluid overload.

Vocal Cord Dysfunction (VCD): Paradoxical adduction of vocal cords during inspiration, causing inspiratory stridor and dyspnea, often triggered by exercise. PFTs may show inspiratory flow limitation, direct laryngoscopy is diagnostic.

Bronchiectasis: Chronic cough, sputum, localized crackles, and recurrent infections.

Foreign Body Aspiration: Acute onset, especially in children, with unilateral wheezing or cough.

Chronic Obstructive Pulmonary Disease (COPD):

Key Features: Progressive, largely irreversible airflow limitation due to chronic bronchitis and/or emphysema. Characterized by chronic cough, sputum production, and exertional dyspnea, typically in middle-aged or older individuals with a significant smoking history.

Differentials:

Asthma: Younger age, significant reversibility on PFTs, atopy, nocturnal symptoms.

Congestive Heart Failure: Dyspnea is prominent, but with cardiac signs/ symptoms, normal PFTs, and positive cardiac markers.

Bronchiectasis: High-resolution CT (HRCT) typically shows bronchial wall thickening and dilatation.

Alpha-1 Antitrypsin Deficiency: Causes early-onset emphysema, especially in non-smokers or those with a small smoking history, often with a basal predominance on imaging.

Pneumonia:

Key Features: Acute infection of the lung parenchyma, presenting with fever, cough (often productive), dyspnea, and pleuritic chest pain.

Physical exam may reveal localized crackles, egophony, or dullness to percussion.

Differentials:

Acute Bronchitis: Cough, but typically without systemic signs of infection (high fever, significant dyspnea) or infiltrates on CXR.

Congestive Heart Failure: Pulmonary edema can mimic pneumonia on CXR (diffuse infiltrates vs. lobar consolidation), but with cardiac findings and elevated BNP.

Pulmonary Embolism: Can cause fever and lung infiltrates (Hampton's hump, Westermark sign), but with characteristic sudden onset dyspnea and risk factors.

Atelectasis: Lung collapse causing crackles and dullness, distinct from infection.

Lung Cancer: Can present as persistent or recurrent "pneumonia" that fails to resolve with antibiotics.

Tuberculosis (TB):

Key Features: Chronic granulomatous infection, primarily affecting the lungs. Presents with chronic cough, weight loss, night sweats, fever, fatigue, and sometimes hemoptysis. Risk factors include immunocompromised status (HIV), close contact, and travel to endemic areas.

Differentials:

Lung Cancer: Shares many symptoms (cough, weight loss, hemoptysis, lung lesions). Differentiated by biopsy.

Atypical Mycobacterial Infections: Similar clinical and radiological presentation, requiring specialized cultures for differentiation.

Fungal Infections (e.g., Histoplasmosis, Coccidioidomycosis): Endemic to certain regions, can cause granulomatous lung disease mimicking TB.

Sarcoidosis: Non-caseating granulomas, can affect lungs and other organs, but negative TB tests and characteristic imaging findings.

Interstitial Lung Disease (ILD):

Key Features: A heterogeneous group of disorders characterized by inflammation and/or fibrosis of the lung interstitium. Presents with progressive exertional dyspnea, dry cough, and often inspiratory crackles ("Velcro rales") on auscultation. Digital clubbing may be present.

Differentials:

Congestive Heart Failure: Pulmonary edema can cause dyspnea and crackles, but cardiac workup is key.

COPD: Obstructive pattern on PFTs, smoking history.

Sarcoidosis: Can cause ILD, but often with involvement of lymph nodes, skin, eyes, and elevated ACE levels.

Hypersensitivity Pneumonitis: ILD caused by exposure to organic dusts, often with acute exacerbations and environmental triggers.

Drug-Induced Lung Disease: Numerous medications can cause ILD (e.g., amiodarone, methotrexate, bleomycin).

Pulmonary Hypertension (PH):

Key Features: Elevated blood pressure in the pulmonary arteries, leading to progressive dyspnea, fatigue, chest pain, and syncope. Signs of right ventricular failure (JVD, peripheral edema) may be present in advanced disease.

Differentials:

Left Heart Disease: The most common cause of PH (Group 2), requiring echocardiography to assess left ventricular function.

Chronic Lung Disease: PH due to hypoxemia and vascular remodeling (Group 3, e.g., COPD, ILD).

Chronic Thromboembolic Pulmonary Hypertension (CTEPH): PH due to unresolved pulmonary emboli (Group 4). CT pulmonary angiography (CTPA) or V/Q scan is crucial.

Primary Pulmonary Arterial Hypertension (PAH): Idiopathic or inherited (Group 1), a diagnosis of exclusion.

Lung Cancer:

Key Features: Malignant growth in the lungs, often presenting with persistent cough, hemoptysis, weight loss, dyspnea, chest pain, and recurrent infections. Smoking is the leading risk factor.

Differentials:

Tuberculosis: Shares many symptoms and radiographic findings. Differentiated by microbiology and biopsy.

Benign Lung Nodules: Common findings, but require careful follow-up and sometimes biopsy to rule out malignancy (especially with growth or high-risk features).

Chronic Pneumonia/Lung Abscess: Can mimic cancer radiologically, but typically resolve with antibiotics. Persistence is a red flag.

Metastatic Disease: Lung involvement by cancers originating elsewhere.

Diagnostic Approaches: A Systematic Inquiry

A judicious selection of diagnostic tools, guided by the clinical presentation, is essential for efficient and accurate diagnosis.

History and Physical Examination: The cornerstone. Detailed symptom analysis (onset, duration, character, aggravating/alleviating factors, associated symptoms), risk factors (smoking, occupational/ environmental exposures, travel, family history), comorbidities, medications. Physical exam focuses on vital signs, respiratory effort, auscultation (wheezes, crackles, rub), percussion, palpation, and signs of systemic disease (clubbing, cyanosis, peripheral edema, lymphadenopathy).

Imaging Studies:

Chest X-ray (CXR): Often the first-line imaging. Useful for detecting pneumonia, pneumothorax, effusion, severe COPD changes (hyperinflation), and gross masses. Limited for subtle interstitial changes or early lesions.

Computed Tomography (CT) Scan: Offers superior anatomical detail.

Standard CT Chest: For masses, mediastinal pathology, complex effusions.

High-Resolution CT (HRCT): Gold standard for interstitial lung diseases, bronchiectasis, and emphysema.

CT Angiography (CTPA): Diagnostic for pulmonary embolism.

Pulmonary Function Tests (PFTs): Crucial for evaluating lung mechanics and gas exchange.

Spirometry: Measures FEV1, FVC, and FEV1/FVC ratio, differentiating obstructive from restrictive patterns and assessing bronchodilator responsiveness (for asthma).

Lung Volumes (Plethysmography): Measures total lung capacity (TLC), functional residual capacity (FRC), and residual volume (RV), confirming restrictive defects and assessing hyperinflation.

Diffusion Capacity for Carbon Monoxide (DLCO): Measures gas exchange efficiency, reduced in ILD, emphysema, and pulmonary vascular disease.

Laboratory Tests:

Complete Blood Count (CBC): Anemia (dyspnea), leukocytosis (infection).

Inflammatory Markers (CRP, Procalcitonin): Infection, inflammation.

D-dimer: Screening for PE (high negative predictive value).

Sputum Culture and Sensitivity, Acid-Fast Bacilli (AFB) Smear/Culture, PCR: For bacterial, mycobacterial, and fungal infections.

Arterial Blood Gases (ABGs): Assess oxygenation and ventilation status.

Brain Natriuretic Peptide (BNP): Differentiates cardiac from pulmonary dyspnea.

Autoimmune Panel: For connective tissue disease-associated ILD or vasculitis.

Microbiological and Histopathological Studies:

Bronchoscopy with Bronchoalveolar Lavage (BAL) and/or Biopsy: Allows direct visualization, collection of fluid for microbiology/cytology, and tissue for histology. Useful for diagnosing infections, malignancies, and ILD.

Thoracentesis: Drainage and analysis of pleural fluid for effusions.

Lung Biopsy (Surgical/Transbronchial): When less invasive methods are inconclusive, particularly for ILD or malignancy.

Cardiac Evaluation:

Electrocardiogram (ECG): Rule out cardiac ischemia, identify arrhythmias, signs of right heart strain (in PE/PH).

Echocardiogram: Assesses cardiac structure and function, crucial for differentiating cardiac vs. pulmonary dyspnea, and for evaluating pulmonary hypertension.

Nuclear Medicine:

Ventilation-Perfusion (V/Q) Scan: Alternative to CTPA for PE diagnosis, particularly when CT contrast is contraindicated (e.g., renal failure, severe contrast allergy).

Summary of the table – Key Differentiators

Symptom / Disease	Key Features	Diagnostic Approaches	Key Differentiating Factors
Acute Cough	< 3 weeks; viral URI, acute bronchitis, pertussis, pneumonia	Clinical exam, CXR (pneumonia), Pertussis PCR	Fever/systemic illness, focal infiltrates (pneumonia); paroxysmal cough + whoop (pertussis)
Chronic Cough	> 8 weeks; UACS, Asthma, GERD, ACEI	PFTs, HRCT, pH monitoring, ENT exam, ACEI trial off	Wheeze + reversibility (Asthma); postnasal drip (UACS); heartburn/ nocturnal cough (GERD); ACEI use
Dyspnea (Cardiac)	Orthopnea, PND, edema, JVD, S3 gallop	ECG, Echo, BNP, CXR (cardiomegaly, Kerley B lines)	Cardiac dysfunction, diuretic response, no primary lung findings
Dyspnea (Pulmonary)	Wheeze, crackles, cough, hypoxemia	PFTs, CXR/CT, ABG	Obstructive vs restrictive PFTs; emphysema, fibrosis, infiltrates on imaging
Hemoptysis	Blood in sputum (streaked → massive)	CXR/CT, Bronchoscopy, Sputum culture, Coagulation studies	TB (night sweats, weight loss), Cancer (smoking, mass), Bronchiectasis, PE, vasculitis
Pleuritic Chest Pain	Sharp, stabbing, worse with inspiration/cough	CXR, CTPA (PE), D-dimer, ECG/ Echo	Pneumonia (fever, cough); Pneumothorax/PE (sudden + dyspnea); pleural rub (pleurisy)
Asthma	Episodic wheeze, cough, dyspnea, chest tightness; reversible obstruction	Spirometry + BD response, FeNO, Allergy testing	Variability, reversibility, atopy, bronchodilator response

COPD	Chronic cough, sputum, exertional dyspnea; irreversible obstruction; smoking	Spirometry (post-BD FEV1/FVC <0.7), HRCT	Smoking, older age, fixed obstruction, emphysema/bronchitis features
Pneumonia	Fever, productive cough, pleuritic pain, localized crackles	CXR infiltrate, Sputum & blood cultures, CRP/Procalcitonin	Acute onset, focal infiltrate, microbiology confirmation
Tuberculosis	Chronic cough, weight loss, fever, night sweats, hemoptysis	AFB smear/culture, GeneXpert, IGRA, CXR/CT (apical lesions, cavities)	Risk factors, positive microbiology, cavitary apical lesions
Interstitial Lung Disease (ILD)	Progressive dyspnea, dry cough, “Velcro” crackles, clubbing	HRCT (reticular, honeycombing, GGO), PFTs (restriction, ↓DLCO), Biopsy	Restrictive PFTs, HRCT patterns, multisystem associations
Pulmonary Hypertension	Dyspnea, fatigue, syncope, chest pain; RV failure signs	Echo, Right heart cath, CTPA (CTEPH), PFTs, sleep study	Elevated PA pressures, classification into pre-/post-capillary causes
Lung Cancer	Persistent cough, hemoptysis, weight loss, chest pain, smoker	CXR/CT (mass/nodule), PET, Bronchoscopy/biopsy, Cytology	Smoking, progressive lesions on imaging, positive pathology

Key Takeaways (Clinical Pearls)

Systematic Approach: Always start with a thorough history and physical. Nuances in symptom description are invaluable.

Red Flags: Be vigilant for "red flag" symptoms that demand urgent investigation: acute severe dyspnea, massive hemoptysis, unresolving pneumonia, new-onset chest pain, significant unintentional weight loss, or persistent symptoms in a high-risk individual (e.g., smoker).

Context Matters: Patient age, smoking history, occupational exposures, travel history, comorbidities, and medication list significantly narrow the differential.

Iterative Process: Diagnosis is often an iterative process. Initial tests may guide further, more specific investigations.

Multidisciplinary Input: Complex cases, especially ILD or lung cancer, often benefit from a multidisciplinary team approach involving pulmonologists, radiologists, pathologists, and thoracic surgeons.

Don't Forget the Basics: Simple tests like a CXR or a sputum sample can still provide game-changing information.

Summary

The differential diagnosis of respiratory diseases is a complex but rewarding endeavor. By systematically evaluating key symptoms like cough, dyspnea, hemoptysis, and chest pain, and understanding the distinct clinical profiles of common pulmonary conditions, clinicians can navigate the diagnostic landscape with greater precision. Integrating a comprehensive history and physical examination with targeted diagnostic investigations, ranging from basic imaging and laboratory tests to advanced PFTs, bronchoscopy, and specialized CT scans, is paramount. The goal is not merely to identify a disease, but to understand its specific characteristics, enabling effective management and improved patient outcomes. A vigilant eye for red flags and a willingness to explore beyond the obvious are the hallmarks of astute clinical practice in pulmonology.

Bibliography and Further Reading

Irwin, R. S., Rosenow, E. C., & Braman, S. S. (1990). Cough: a comprehensive review. Chest, 98(2), 220S-226S. (Classic, but still foundational for cough classification).

Khurana, R., & Gupta, A. (2020). Pulmonary Embolism. StatPearls [Internet]. Treasure Island (FL): StatPearls Publishing. (Recent review on PE diagnosis and management).

American Thoracic Society. (2019). An Official ATS/ERS/JRS/ALAT Clinical Practice Guideline: Diagnosis of Idiopathic Pulmonary Fibrosis. American Journal of Respiratory and Critical Care Medicine, 200(5), e126-e152. (Key guideline for ILD diagnosis, including HRCT and biopsy recommendations).

Global Initiative for Chronic Obstructive Lung Disease (GOLD). (2023). Global Strategy for the Diagnosis, Management, and Prevention of Chronic Obstructive Pulmonary Disease. (Annual update providing comprehensive guidance on COPD).

Global Initiative for Asthma (GINA). (2023). Global Strategy for Asthma Management and Prevention. (Annual update for asthma diagnosis and management).

World Health Organization. (2023). Global Tuberculosis Report 2023. (Provides an overview of TB epidemiology and updated diagnostic approaches).

Heschl, S., et al. (2021). The role of lung cancer in the differential diagnosis of chronic cough. Journal of Thoracic Disease, 13(7), 4059–4070. (Discusses lung cancer as a cause of chronic cough).

McLaughlin, V. V., et al. (2019). ESC/ERS Guidelines for the diagnosis and treatment of pulmonary hypertension. European Respiratory Journal, 53(1), 1801913. (Comprehensive guidelines for PH diagnosis and management).

Chapter Three

Differential Diagnosis of Acute and Chronic Abdominal Pain

Dr. Arivarasan

Introduction

Abdominal pain is an exceptionally common complaint presenting to healthcare professionals across all settings, from primary care clinics to emergency departments. It is estimated that a significant proportion of the population will experience abdominal pain at some point in their lives, with a considerable number seeking medical attention. The diverse nature of abdominal pain, ranging from mild and self-limiting to severe and life-threatening, necessitates a robust understanding of its differential diagnosis. Accurate diagnosis is paramount, as it dictates timely and appropriate management, ultimately influencing patient outcomes and minimizing morbidity and mortality.

This comprehensive article aims to provide a detailed exploration of the differential diagnosis of both acute and chronic abdominal pain. We will delve into the broad spectrum of potential Etiologies, emphasizing the importance of recognizing key clinical presentations, employing systematic diagnostic approaches, and understanding the nuances that differentiate various conditions. Furthermore, we will provide a comparative summary highlighting the distinctions and overlaps between acute and chronic abdominal pain syndromes, outline key takeaways for clinicians, and conclude with a concise summary. To ensure the information is current and evidence-based, a comprehensive bibliography incorporating recent research will be included.

Understanding Abdominal Pain: Anatomy, Physiology, and Pain Pathways

To effectively approach the differential diagnosis, a foundational understanding of abdominal anatomy, relevant physiology, and pain pathways is essential. The abdomen is a complex cavity containing a multitude of organs derived from various embryological origins, each with distinct innervation patterns. This anatomical complexity contributes to the diagnostic challenge of abdominal pain.

1. Anatomical Regions and Organ Systems:

The abdomen is conventionally divided into nine regions (right hypochondriac, epigastric, left hypochondriac, right lumbar, umbilical, left lumbar, right iliac, hypogastric, and left iliac) or four quadrants (right upper quadrant (RUQ), left upper quadrant (LUQ), right lower quadrant (RLQ), and left lower quadrant (LLQ)). While these divisions are useful for localization, it is crucial to remember that pain perception can be referred and visceral pain often poorly localized.

The abdominal cavity houses organ systems vital for numerous bodily functions:

- Gastrointestinal System: Esophagus, stomach, small intestine (duodenum, jejunum, ileum), large intestine (cecum, colon, rectum), and anus. These organs are primarily involved in digestion, absorption, and elimination.
- Hepatobiliary System: Liver, gallbladder, and biliary tree. Crucial for metabolism, bile production, and storage.
- Pancreas: Both exocrine (digestive enzymes) and endocrine (hormones like insulin and glucagon) functions.
- Spleen: Part of the lymphatic system, involved in immune function and blood filtration.
- Urinary System: Kidneys, ureters, bladder, and urethra. Responsible for waste excretion and fluid balance.
- Reproductive System: Ovaries, fallopian tubes, and uterus in females; testes, epididymis, vas deferens, prostate, and seminal

vesicles in males. Involved in reproduction and hormone production.

- Vascular System: Abdominal aorta, inferior vena cava, and their branches. Supply blood to the abdominal organs and systemic circulation.
- Musculoskeletal System: Abdominal wall muscles and bones of the lower ribs and pelvis. Provide support and movement.
- Nervous System: Autonomic nervous system (sympathetic and parasympathetic) and somatic nervous system innervate abdominal organs and structures.

2. Pain Pathways: Visceral, Somatic, and Referred Pain:

Understanding the different types of pain pathways is crucial for interpreting patient symptoms and narrowing the differential diagnosis. Abdominal pain can be broadly categorized into visceral, somatic, and referred pain.

- Visceral Pain: Originates from the abdominal viscera and is mediated by visceral afferent nerve fibers. These fibers are sensitive to distention, contraction, ischemia, and inflammation, but relatively insensitive to cutting, burning, or sharp stimuli. Visceral pain is typically described as dull, crampy, achy, or gnawing, and it is often poorly localized due to the sparse and diffuse innervation of visceral organs. Pain from midline structures (e.g., stomach, small bowel) tends to be felt in the midline epigastrium, periumbilical region, or hypogastrium, while pain from paired organs (e.g., kidneys) may be felt more laterally in the flanks.
- Somatic (Parietal) Pain: Arises from the parietal peritoneum, abdominal wall muscles, and skin. Somatic afferent nerve fibers are more numerous and well-localized compared to visceral fibers. Somatic pain is generally sharp, well-localized, and intensifies with movement or coughing. Irritation of the parietal

peritoneum, such as in appendicitis or peritonitis, elicits somatic pain.

- Referred Pain: Pain felt in a location distant from the source of the pain stimuli. It occurs because visceral and somatic afferent nerve fibers converge in the spinal cord and brain, leading to misinterpretation of the pain origin by the brain. Common examples include:
    - Right shoulder pain referred from gallbladder disease (phrenic nerve irritation).
    - Left shoulder pain referred from splenic rupture or irritation of the diaphragm.
    - Back pain referred from pancreatic disease or aortic aneurysm.
    - Groin pain referred from renal colic.

Differentiating Acute and Chronic Abdominal Pain:

The temporal characteristic of abdominal pain, whether acute or chronic, significantly influences the differential diagnosis and diagnostic approach.

1. Acute Abdominal Pain:

Acute abdominal pain is generally defined as pain of recent onset, typically lasting less than 7 days. It often presents abruptly and may be severe, requiring prompt assessment and intervention. Acute abdominal pain frequently indicates a new pathological process and can be a symptom of a surgical emergency or a medical condition requiring immediate attention.

2. Chronic Abdominal Pain:

Chronic abdominal pain is defined as pain that persists for more than three months, either continuously or intermittently. It is often less severe than acute pain but can significantly impact quality of life. Chronic abdominal pain presents a diagnostic challenge as it can be caused by a wide range of conditions, including organic diseases, functional disorders, and psychological factors.

Acute Abdominal Pain: Differential Diagnosis, Key Presentations, and Diagnostic Approaches

Acute abdominal pain, often termed the "acute abdomen," is a critical clinical entity demanding rapid and systematic evaluation to exclude life-threatening conditions. The differential diagnosis is broad and encompasses a diverse range of etiologies.

I. Etiologies of Acute Abdominal Pain:

Acute abdominal pain can be categorized based on the organ system involved or by the underlying pathological mechanism.

A. Gastrointestinal Causes:

- Appendicitis: Inflammation of the vermiform appendix, the most common surgical emergency in the abdomen.
    - Key Presentations:
        - Initial Presentation: Vague periumbilical pain (visceral pain).
        - Later Presentation: Pain migrates to the RLQ (somatic pain due to parietal peritoneal irritation – McBurney's point tenderness).
        - Anorexia, nausea, vomiting, low-grade fever common.
        - Rovsing's sign (RLQ pain with LLQ palpation), Obturator sign (pain with internal rotation of flexed hip), Psoas sign (pain with hip extension) may be present.
    - Diagnostic Approaches:
        - History and Physical Examination: Crucial for initial assessment.

- Laboratory Tests: Complete blood count (CBC) (leucocytosis with neutrophilia), C-reactive protein (CRP) may be elevated. Urinalysis to rule out urinary tract infection (UTI).
- Imaging:
  - CT scan of the Abdomen and Pelvis with IV contrast: Gold standard for diagnosis in adults, high sensitivity and specificity.
  - Ultrasound: Useful in children and pregnant women to avoid radiation exposure; operator-dependent and less sensitive than CT in adults.
  - Plain Abdominal Radiograph: Limited role, may show fecalith in appendix, but not diagnostic of appendicitis.

- Acute Diverticulitis: Inflammation and infection of diverticula (small pouches) in the colon, most commonly in the sigmoid colon.
  - Key Presentations:
    - LLQ pain: Typically, gradual onset, constant, and localized to the LLQ.
    - Fever, chills, leucocytosis.
    - Changes in bowel habits (constipation or diarrhea).
    - Nausea and vomiting may be present.
  - Diagnostic Approaches:
    - History and Physical Examination: Palpation reveals LLQ tenderness, guarding, or rigidity.
    - Laboratory Tests: CBC (leucocytosis), CRP elevated.
    - Imaging:
      - CT scan of the Abdomen and Pelvis with IV contrast: Diagnostic imaging modality of choice. Demonstrates

diverticula, colonic wall thickening, peri colonic fat stranding, and abscess formation.
- Colonoscopy/Sigmoidoscopy: Contraindicated in the acute phase due to risk of perforation; performed after resolution to rule out malignancy.

- Intestinal Obstruction: Blockage of the small or large intestine, preventing the normal passage of intestinal contents. Can be mechanical (e.g., adhesions, hernia, tumor) or non-mechanical (e.g., ileus).
  - Key Presentations:
    - Crampy, intermittent abdominal pain: Characterized by waves of pain that coincide with peristaltic rushes.
    - Abdominal distention.
    - Vomiting (especially with proximal obstructions).
    - Obstipation (absence of stool and flatus).
    - High-pitched bowel sounds (early obstruction), absent bowel sounds (late obstruction with ileus).
  - Diagnostic Approaches:
    - History and Physical Examination: Assess for prior surgeries, hernias, and abdominal distention.
    - Laboratory Tests: Electrolyte imbalances, dehydration markers.
    - Imaging:
      - Plain Abdominal Radiograph (Upright and Supine): Shows dilated loops of bowel, air-fluid levels (step-ladder appearance). Can differentiate small bowel from large bowel obstruction.
      - CT scan of the Abdomen and Pelvis with IV contrast: Identifies the level and cause of obstruction, and can detect complications (e.g., ischemia, perforation).

        - Contrast Enema: May be useful in colonic obstruction to identify the level of obstruction and may be therapeutic in some cases of sigmoid volvulus.

- Perforation of a Viscus: Rupture of a hollow organ, such as the stomach, duodenum, colon, or gallbladder, leading to leakage of contents into the peritoneal cavity. Common causes include peptic ulcer disease, diverticulitis, appendicitis, trauma.

    - Key Presentations:

        - Sudden onset of severe, agonizing abdominal pain: "Knife-like" pain.
        - Generalized abdominal tenderness and rigidity (board-like abdomen) due to peritonitis.
        - Hypotension, tachycardia, signs of sepsis.
        - Free air under the diaphragm on chest or abdominal radiograph.

    - Diagnostic Approaches:

        - History and Physical Examination: Signs of peritonitis (rebound tenderness, guarding, rigidity).
        - Laboratory Tests: CBC (leucocytosis), electrolyte imbalances, sepsis markers.
        - Imaging:

            - Plain Abdominal Radiograph (Upright Chest or Abdomen): Pneumoperitoneum (free air under the diaphragm) is a hallmark finding.
            - CT scan of the Abdomen and Pelvis with IV contrast: Confirms perforation, identifies the site, and assesses for underlying pathology and complications.

- Gastroenteritis: Inflammation of the stomach and intestines, typically caused by viral or bacterial infections.

- Key Presentations:
    - Diffuse, crampy abdominal pain.
    - Nausea, vomiting, diarrhea (may be watery or bloody).
    - Fever, myalgia, headache.
    - Dehydration.
- Diagnostic Approaches:
    - History and Physical Examination: Focus on travel history, dietary history, sick contacts. Assess hydration status.
    - Laboratory Tests: Usually not necessary for mild cases. Stool studies (fecal leukocytes, ova and parasites, culture, PCR for specific pathogens) may be indicated in severe, persistent, or bloody diarrhea.
    - Imaging: Generally, not required unless suspecting complications or alternative diagnoses.

- Mesenteric Ischemia: Reduced blood flow to the small intestine and colon, leading to bowel ischemia and infarction. Can be acute (embolus, thrombus) or chronic. Acute mesenteric ischemia is a surgical emergency.
    - Key Presentations:
        - Severe, diffuse abdominal pain: "Pain out of proportion to physical exam findings" is a classic, but not always present, feature.
        - Nausea, vomiting, diarrhea (may be bloody).
        - Abdominal distention.
        - Late findings: signs of peritonitis, septic shock.
        - Risk factors: atrial fibrillation, atherosclerosis, hypercoagulable states, recent cardiac surgery.

- Diagnostic Approaches:
  - History and Physical Examination: Assess for risk factors and signs of shock.
  - Laboratory Tests: Lactic acidosis, leucocytosis, elevated amylase, phosphate, D-dimer.
  - Imaging:
    - CT Angiography of the Abdomen and Pelvis: Diagnostic test of choice. Visualizes mesenteric arteries and veins to identify occlusion or stenosis.
    - Mesenteric Angiography (Catheter-based): Gold standard for diagnosis and allows for potential intervention (thrombolysis, angioplasty).

B. Hepatobiliary Causes:

- Acute Cholecystitis: Inflammation of the gallbladder, usually caused by gallstones obstructing the cystic duct.
  - Key Presentations:
    - RUQ pain: Sudden onset, constant, severe, often radiating to the right shoulder or back (referred pain).
    - Nausea, vomiting, anorexia.
    - Fever, chills, leucocytosis.
    - Murphy's sign (inspiratory arrest with RUQ palpation under the costal margin) is often positive.
  - Diagnostic Approaches:
    - History and Physical Examination: RUQ tenderness, Murphy's sign.
    - Laboratory Tests: Leucocytosis, elevated alkaline phosphatase, bilirubin (mild elevation), liver enzymes (mildly elevated).

- Imaging:
    - Right Upper Quadrant Ultrasound: Initial imaging modality of choice. Detects gallstones, gallbladder wall thickening, pericholecystic fluid, and sonographic Murphy's sign.
    - HIDA Scan (Hepatobiliary Iminodiacetic Acid Scan): Used if ultrasound is inconclusive. Demonstrates cystic duct obstruction.
    - CT scan of the Abdomen and Pelvis with IV contrast: May be used if ultrasound is non-diagnostic or to rule out other conditions.

- Ascending Cholangitis: Infection of the biliary tree, usually due to biliary obstruction (often gallstones) and bacterial overgrowth. Life-threatening emergency.
    - Key Presentations:
        - Charcot's Triad: RUQ pain, fever, jaundice.
        - Reynold's Pentad: Charcot's triad plus shock and altered mental status (indicates severe sepsis).
        - RUQ tenderness.
    - Diagnostic Approaches:
        - History and Physical Examination: Assess for Charcot's triad and Reynold's pentad.
        - Laboratory Tests: Leucocytosis, elevated bilirubin (direct hyperbilirubinemia), alkaline phosphatase, liver enzymes. Blood cultures to identify causative organism.
        - Imaging:
            - RUQ Ultrasound: May show

Differential Diagnosis of Constipation

Introduction

Constipation, a ubiquitous gastrointestinal complaint, affects individuals across all ages and demographics, significantly impacting their quality of life. While often dismissed as a mere inconvenience, constipation is a complex symptom with a diverse range of underlying etiologies, from benign functional disorders to serious organic pathologies.

The definition of constipation, often surprisingly subjective, generally revolves around infrequent bowel movements, difficult passage of stool, and a constellation of associated symptoms like straining, incomplete evacuation, and abdominal discomfort. However, relying solely on frequency is insufficient, as "normal" bowel habits vary widely among individuals. The Rome IV criteria, a globally recognized diagnostic framework, provides a more nuanced definition, focusing on symptom-based criteria rather than solely on bowel movement frequency, thus capturing the subjective experience of constipation more accurately.

The importance of a robust differential diagnosis in constipation cannot be overstated. Accurately identifying the underlying cause is paramount for effective management, preventing unnecessary investigations, and most importantly, ruling out serious conditions that may present with constipation as a primary symptom. Misdiagnosis or a superficial approach to constipation can lead to delayed treatment of underlying medical conditions, inappropriate management strategies, and persistent patient suffering. This chapter delves into the multifaceted landscape of constipation, systematically exploring key presentations, diagnostic approaches, and the crucial process of differential diagnosis to empower clinicians and patients alike in navigating this common yet complex clinical challenge. We will dissect the various categories of constipation, from functional disorders to secondary causes stemming from medications, systemic illnesses, and structural abnormalities, providing a comprehensive guide for differentiating between them.

Furthermore, we will outline the diagnostic algorithms and tools available to aid in this process, culminating in a comparative summary and key takeaways to solidify understanding and facilitate practical application in clinical settings.

Key Presentations of Constipation

Constipation is not a monolithic entity. It manifests in a spectrum of presentations, each providing valuable clues to the underlying cause. Understanding these nuanced presentations is the first step in navigating the differential diagnosis. We can categorize these presentations based on several key aspects:

1. Onset and Duration:

- Acute Constipation: A sudden change in bowel habits, typically occurring over days to weeks, often with a clear precipitating factor like dietary changes, medications, travel, or acute illness. While often transient, acute constipation can be alarming and requires careful evaluation to rule out serious causes, particularly bowel obstruction or acute systemic illness. Red flag symptoms such as severe abdominal pain, vomiting, or rectal bleeding accompanying acute constipation warrant prompt medical attention.
- Chronic Constipation: Constipation persisting for three months or longer, fulfilling the Rome IV criteria for chronic constipation. Chronic constipation is frequently categorized as functional, but secondary causes need to be meticulously considered. The insidious nature of chronic constipation can sometimes lead to delayed diagnosis of underlying conditions.

2. Stool Characteristics:

- Bristol Stool Chart: This validated visual aid categorizes stool into seven types, ranging from hard, separate lumps (Type 1) to watery, no solid pieces (Type 7). Types 1 and 2 are indicative of constipation, representing hard and lumpy stools that are difficult to pass. The Bristol Stool Chart is a simple yet powerful tool for standardizing the description of stool consistency and can be effectively used in patient interviews and clinical documentation.

- Hard Stools: Characterized by types 1 and 2 on the Bristol Stool Chart, hard stools are often associated with straining, pain during defecation, and a sense of incomplete evacuation. They indicate prolonged colonic transit time, allowing for excessive water reabsorption in the colon, leading to dehydration of the faecal matter.
- Narrow Stools (Pencil-thin stools): While not always indicative of constipation itself, a persistent change to narrow stools, especially in conjunction with other constipation symptoms, can be a concerning sign. It may suggest a distal obstruction in the rectum or sigmoid colon, such as a stricture or colorectal cancer. This warrants further investigation, particularly in older individuals or those with risk factors for colorectal cancer.
- Mucoid Stools: The presence of mucus in the stool, while not directly defining constipation, can be associated with certain subtypes of constipation, particularly Irritable Bowel Syndrome with Constipation (IBS-C). It may reflect underlying intestinal inflammation or altered gut motility.

3. Associated Symptoms:

- Abdominal Pain and Bloating: Commonly reported in constipation, ranging from mild discomfort to significant pain. Bloating, a subjective sensation of abdominal distention, is also frequently experienced. The nature and location of pain can offer clues; for instance, diffuse, crampy pain may be more suggestive of functional constipation or IBS-C, while localized or progressively worsening pain might indicate structural issues.
- Straining during Defecation: Excessive effort required to pass stool, often accompanied by a feeling of incomplete evacuation.

Significant straining can contribute to anorectal complications like haemorrhoids and anal fissures. It is a hallmark symptom of both slow transit constipation and pelvic floor dysfunction.

- Sense of Incomplete Evacuation: The feeling that the bowels are not fully emptied despite defecation. This is a prominent symptom in pelvic floor dysfunction and can contribute to significant patient distress.
- Rectal Bleeding: While often minor and associated with haemorrhoids or anal fissures secondary to straining, rectal bleeding accompanying constipation should never be dismissed. It can be a red flag for more serious conditions like colorectal cancer or inflammatory bowel disease, especially if it is persistent, bright red, or associated with other alarm symptoms.
- Weight Loss: Unexplained weight loss in the context of constipation is a significant red flag. It can be indicative of underlying malignancy, malabsorption syndromes, or systemic illnesses. Prompt investigation is crucial in such cases.
- Nausea and Vomiting: These symptoms, particularly in acute constipation, can suggest bowel obstruction or other serious gastrointestinal pathology. They warrant urgent medical evaluation.
- Fatigue and Lethargy: Chronic constipation can contribute to systemic symptoms like fatigue and lethargy, possibly due to gut dysbiosis, inflammation, or altered nutrient absorption.

4. Frequency and Timing of Bowel Movements:

- Infrequent Bowel Movements: Defined by fewer than three bowel movements per week according to the Rome IV criteria. While frequency alone is not sufficient for diagnosis, it is a key element of the classic definition of constipation.
- Diurnal Pattern: Understanding the typical timing of bowel movements can be helpful. Some individuals experience constipation primarily in the mornings, while others throughout

the day. Changes in the usual diurnal pattern may suggest altered colonic motility or external factors influencing bowel habits.

5. Response to Laxatives:

- Laxative Responsiveness: How a patient responds to different types of laxatives (bulk-forming, osmotic, stimulant) can provide insights into the underlying mechanism of their constipation. For instance, poor response to stimulant laxatives might suggest slow transit constipation, while lack of response to bulk-forming agents might imply pelvic floor dysfunction.
- Laxative Dependence: Chronic laxative use, particularly stimulant laxatives, can paradoxically worsen constipation over time by leading to colonic inertia (reduced colonic motility) or electrolyte imbalances. This is an important aspect to assess in patients with chronic constipation.

By meticulously analysing these key presentations – onset, stool characteristics, associated symptoms, frequency, and laxative response – clinicians can begin to narrow down the differential diagnosis and tailor their investigative approach effectively.

Diagnostic Approaches to Constipation

A systematic approach to diagnosing constipation is essential, moving from initial history and physical examination to targeted investigations based on clinical suspicion. The diagnostic process aims to differentiate between functional constipation and secondary constipation stemming from underlying medical conditions.

1. Comprehensive History and Physical Examination:

- Detailed Symptom Assessment: A thorough history is the cornerstone of constipation diagnosis. This includes:
    - Detailed Description of Constipation: Onset, duration, frequency of bowel movements, stool consistency (using

Bristol Stool Chart if possible), straining, sense of incomplete evacuation, presence of mucus or blood.

- Associated Symptoms: Abdominal pain, bloating, nausea, vomiting, weight loss, fatigue.
- Bowel Habit History: Normal bowel habits before onset of constipation, changes in bowel habits, factors that worsen or relieve symptoms.
- Dietary History: Fiber intake, fluid intake, dietary changes, dietary restrictions.
- Medication History: Prescription medications, over-the-counter medications, supplements, and laxative use (type, frequency, duration). Particular attention should be paid to medications known to cause constipation, such as opioids, anticholinergics, calcium channel blockers, iron supplements, and certain antidepressants.
- Past Medical History: Existing medical conditions, particularly endocrine disorders (hypothyroidism, diabetes), neurological disorders (Parkinson's disease, multiple sclerosis, spinal cord injury), gastrointestinal disorders (irritable bowel syndrome, inflammatory bowel disease), psychiatric conditions (depression, anxiety, eating disorders), and history of colorectal cancer or surgery.
- Surgical History: Previous abdominal or pelvic surgeries that might have impacted bowel function.
- Social History: Lifestyle factors, including physical activity level, stress levels, travel history, and access to toilet facilities.
- Family History: Family history of colorectal cancer, inflammatory bowel disease, or other gastrointestinal disorders.
- Psychosocial Assessment: Assessing for psychological stressors, anxiety, depression, and history of abuse can be important, as psychological factors can significantly influence bowel function.

    - Review of Systems: A general review of systems to identify potential systemic illnesses that may manifest with constipation.

- Physical Examination: A focused physical examination should include:
    - General Appearance: Assessing for signs of systemic illness, such as weight loss, pallor, or fatigue.
    - Abdominal Examination:
        - Inspection: Distention, scars, visible peristalsis.
        - Auscultation: Bowel sounds (presence, character, frequency – hypoactive bowel sounds may be present in constipation, but absence can indicate ileus or obstruction).
        - Percussion: Tympany (indicating gas accumulation) or dullness (suggesting masses or organomegaly).
        - Palpation: Tenderness, masses, organomegaly, guarding, and rebound tenderness (signs of peritonitis, a surgical emergency that can mimic constipation in early stages).
    - Digital Rectal Examination (DRE): Crucial for assessing:
        - Anal Sphincter Tone: To evaluate for hypertonicity (pelvic floor dysfunction) or hypotonicity (neurological issues).
        - Rectal Vault: Presence of stool impaction, masses, or tenderness.
        - Perianal Area: Haemorrhoids, fissures, skin tags, and signs of inflammation.
        - Sensation: Perianal sensation to assess for neurological deficits.
        - Pelvic Floor Function (during simulated defecation): Paradoxical puborectalis contraction or inadequate relaxation suggests pelvic floor dyssynergia.

2. Red Flag (Alarm) Symptoms:

Identifying red flag symptoms is critical to rule out serious organic pathology and guide urgent investigations. These symptoms warrant prompt medical attention and further evaluation, often including colonoscopy and imaging studies:

- Rectal Bleeding: Especially bright red blood, persistent bleeding, or blood mixed with stool (haematochezia).
- Unexplained Weight Loss: Significant unintentional weight loss in conjunction with constipation.
- Family History of Colorectal Cancer or Inflammatory Bowel Disease: Increased risk of these conditions.
- New Onset Constipation in Older Individuals (over 50 years): Higher risk of colorectal cancer.
- Severe or Progressively Worsening Abdominal Pain: Could indicate obstruction, ischemia, or perforation.
- Nausea and Vomiting: Suggestive of bowel obstruction.
- Anaemia (Iron Deficiency Anaemia): May indicate chronic blood loss from colorectal lesions.
- Palpable Abdominal Mass: Could represent a tumor or other intra-abdominal pathology.
- Fever: Suggests infection or inflammatory process.
- Change in Stool Caliber (Pencil-thin stools): May indicate distal obstruction.
- Nocturnal Symptoms: Symptoms that wake the patient at night are less likely to be functional and more suggestive of organic disease, such as inflammatory bowel disease

3. Initial Investigations (Tier 1):

In the absence of red flag symptoms, initial investigations are often aimed at excluding common secondary causes and assessing for functional constipation.

- Basic Blood Tests:
  - Complete Blood Count (CBC): To check for anaemia (iron deficiency).
  - Electrolytes (Sodium, Potassium, Calcium): Electrolyte imbalances can contribute to constipation. Hypercalcemia, in particular, is a known cause.
  - Thyroid Stimulating Hormone (TSH): To rule out hypothyroidism, a common endocrine cause of constipation.
  - Glucose: To screen for diabetes mellitus, which can cause constipation through autonomic neuropathy.
  - Renal Function Tests (Creatinine, BUN): To assess kidney function, as renal insufficiency can contribute to constipation due to fluid and electrolyte imbalances.
- Stool Tests (Selective):
  - Faecal Occult Blood Test (FOBT) or Faecal Immunochemical Test (FIT): To screen for occult blood in stool, particularly in individuals with risk factors for colorectal cancer, even in the absence of overt rectal bleeding. While not routinely recommended in all cases of constipation, it can be considered in patients over 50 or with risk factors.
  - Stool Calprotectin: If inflammatory bowel disease is suspected, faecal calprotectin can be used as a non-invasive marker of intestinal inflammation. Elevated levels warrant further investigation with colonoscopy.
  - Stool Culture and Ova & Parasites: If infectious etiology is suspected (e.g., acute onset constipation following travel or food poisoning, or immunocompromised individuals), stool cultures and ova & parasites examination may be indicated.

4. Advanced Investigations (Tier 2) – When Indicated:

If red flag symptoms are present, initial investigations are inconclusive, or symptoms persist despite initial management, further investigations are warranted to evaluate for structural, motility, or pelvic floor disorders.

- Structural Imaging:
  - Colonoscopy: The gold standard for evaluating the colon, especially in individuals with red flag symptoms, family history of colorectal cancer, or new-onset constipation in older individuals. Allows for visualization of the colonic mucosa, detection of polyps, tumors, strictures, inflammatory bowel disease, and allows for biopsies.
  - Sigmoidoscopy: A less invasive alternative to colonoscopy, examining only the rectum and sigmoid colon. May be sufficient for screening in lower-risk individuals or for evaluating distal colonic pathology.
  - Barium Enema: Radiographic examination of the colon using barium contrast. Less sensitive than colonoscopy for detecting small lesions but can be useful for evaluating colonic anatomy and obstructing lesions. Less commonly used now with the advent of CT colonography.
  - CT Colonography (Virtual Colonoscopy): A non-invasive imaging technique using CT scan to create 3D images of the colon. Less invasive than colonoscopy but less sensitive for small lesions and does not allow for biopsies. May be an option for patients who are poor candidates for colonoscopy or as a screening tool in specific situations.

Differential Diagnosis of Diarrhea:

Introduction:

Diarrhea, characterized by an increase in stool frequency, fluidity, or volume compared to an individual's usual bowel habits, is a ubiquitous symptom encountered across all ages and demographics. While often a self-limiting inconvenience, diarrhea can also signify serious underlying pathology, ranging from benign viral infections to life-threatening conditions like inflammatory bowel disease or infectious colitis. Navigating the complex landscape of diarrhea requires a systematic approach, a robust understanding of its various etiologies, and a keen ability to differentiate between seemingly similar clinical presentations. This chapter aims to provide a comprehensive guide to the differential diagnosis of diarrhea, equipping clinicians with the necessary tools to effectively evaluate patients, narrow down diagnostic possibilities, and ultimately guide appropriate management strategies.

Key Presentations of Diarrhea:

The clinical presentation of diarrhea is highly variable and depends on the underlying cause, the patient's age and overall health, and the duration of symptoms. Categorizing diarrhea based on its characteristics and associated features is crucial for narrowing the differential diagnosis. We can broadly classify diarrhea based on several key parameters:

1. Duration:

- Acute Diarrhea: Defined as diarrhea lasting less than 14 days, acute diarrhea is most commonly caused by infectious agents, particularly viruses, bacteria, and parasites. Food poisoning, medication side effects, and dietary indiscretions are also common culprits. Acute diarrhea is typically abrupt in onset and often resolves spontaneously within a few days to a week.
- Persistent Diarrhea: This category encompasses diarrhea lasting between 14 and 30 days. Persistent diarrhea may represent prolonged infectious diarrhea, post-infectious irritable bowel syndrome (PI-IBS), or the initial manifestation of chronic diarrheal conditions. Careful evaluation is warranted to exclude ongoing infection or evolving chronic disease.
- Chronic Diarrhea: Diarrhea persisting for more than 30 days is classified as chronic. Chronic diarrhea is less likely to be infectious and more frequently indicates underlying inflammatory conditions (e.g., inflammatory bowel disease,

microscopic colitis), malabsorptive disorders (e.g., celiac disease, pancreatic insufficiency), motility disorders (bile acid diarrhea), or endocrine/metabolic conditions. Chronic diarrhea demands thorough investigation to identify the root cause and guide long-term management.

2. Pathophysiological Mechanisms:

Understanding the underlying pathophysiology of diarrhea is paramount for accurate diagnosis. Diarrhea can be broadly categorized into the following mechanisms:

- Osmotic Diarrhea: This type arises from the presence of poorly absorbed solutes in the intestinal lumen. These solutes draw water into the bowel, increasing stool volume and fluidity. Osmotic diarrhea characteristically ceases when the patient fasts, as the osmotic load is removed. Common causes include:
    - Laxative abuse: Osmotic laxatives (e.g., magnesium salts, lactulose) directly increase luminal osmolality.
    - Malabsorption syndromes: Conditions like lactose intolerance, celiac disease, and short bowel syndrome result in malabsorption of carbohydrates, fats, or other nutrients, leading to an osmotic load in the colon.
    - Tube feeding formulas: Hyperosmolar formulas can induce osmotic diarrhea, especially in patients with impaired digestion or absorption.
    - Certain medications: Sorbitol and mannitol, used as excipients in some medications, can cause osmotic diarrhea.
- Secretory Diarrhea: Characterized by active secretion of electrolytes and water into the intestinal lumen, secretory diarrhea is often high-volume and persists even during fasting. It results from disruption of normal intestinal fluid and electrolyte balance. Common causes include:

  - Enterotoxins: Produced by bacteria like *Vibrio cholerae*, *Escherichia coli*(enterotoxigenic ETEC), and *Clostridium difficile*, these toxins stimulate intestinal chloride secretion, leading to massive watery diarrhea.
  - Hormones: Certain endocrine tumors (e.g., carcinoid tumors, VIPoma's, gastrinomas) secrete hormones that stimulate intestinal secretion.
  - Bile acid malabsorption: Inadequate reabsorption of bile acids in the terminal ileum, often due to ileal resection or disease, can lead to colonic secretion.
  - Congenital secretory diarrhea: Rare inherited disorders affecting intestinal electrolyte transport, such as congenital chloride diarrhea or congenital sodium diarrhea.
  - Certain medications: Stimulant laxatives (e.g., bisacodyl, senna) and some chemotherapeutic agents can induce secretory diarrhea.

- Inflammatory Diarrhea: This type arises from inflammation and damage to the intestinal mucosa. Inflammation disrupts normal absorption and secretion, and the exudation of mucus, blood, and inflammatory cells into the stool contributes to diarrhea. Common causes include:

  - Infectious colitis: Bacteria like *Shigella*, *Salmonella*, *Campylobacter*, *Escherichia coli* (enterohaemorrhagic EHEC), and *Entamoeba histolytica* can invade and inflame the colonic mucosa. *C. difficile* infection, while often secretory, can also cause significant mucosal inflammation (pseudomembranous colitis).
  - Inflammatory bowel disease (IBD): Ulcerative colitis and Crohn's disease are chronic inflammatory conditions of the gastrointestinal tract, often presenting with bloody diarrhea, abdominal pain, and systemic symptoms.

  - Microscopic colitis: Lymphocytic colitis and collagenous colitis are characterized by microscopic inflammation of the colonic mucosa, leading to chronic watery diarrhea, often without gross mucosal abnormalities.
  - Radiation colitis: Radiation therapy to the abdomen or pelvis can cause mucosal damage and inflammation, leading to diarrhea.
  - Ischemic colitis: Reduced blood flow to the colon can result in mucosal ischemia and inflammation, often presenting with abdominal pain and bloody diarrhea, particularly in older individuals with cardiovascular risk factors.

- Motility Diarrhea: Abnormal intestinal motility, either increased or decreased, can contribute to diarrhea. Increased motility can reduce transit time, impairing absorption and leading to diarrhea. Decreased motility can result in bacterial overgrowth, which may also cause diarrhea. Common examples include:

  - Irritable bowel syndrome (IBS): IBS is a functional bowel disorder often characterized by altered bowel habits, including diarrhea-predominant IBS (IBS-D). Abnormal intestinal motility and visceral hypersensitivity are thought to play key roles.
  - Post-vagotomy diarrhea: Vagotomy, historically performed for peptic ulcer disease, can disrupt gastric emptying and intestinal motility, leading to diarrhea.
  - Hyperthyroidism: Excess thyroid hormone can accelerate intestinal motility, contributing to diarrhea.
  - Medications: Prokinetic agents and some antibiotics can increase intestinal motility and induce diarrhea.

3. Stool Characteristics:

Analysing stool characteristics provides valuable clues for differential diagnosis:

- Watery Diarrhea: Suggests secretory or osmotic mechanisms. Large volume watery diarrhea is characteristic of toxin-mediated infections (e.g., cholera, ETEC) and certain endocrine tumors. Small volume watery diarrhea can be seen in IBS-D or early viral gastroenteritis.
- Bloody Diarrhea (Dysentery): Strongly suggestive of inflammatory colitis, typically caused by bacterial infections (e.g., *Shigella*, *Salmonella*, EHEC) or IBD. *E. histolytica* and *C. difficile* can also cause bloody diarrhea.
- Fatty Diarrhea (Steatorrhea): Indicates fat malabsorption and suggests pancreatic insufficiency, celiac disease, small intestinal bacterial overgrowth (SIBO), or bile acid deficiency. Stools are often pale, greasy, foul-smelling, and may float.
- Mucoid Diarrhea: Excessive mucus in the stool can be seen in inflammatory conditions like IBD, infectious colitis (especially *Shigella* and amoebiasis), and IBS.
- Color: While stool color can be influenced by diet, certain colors may suggest specific conditions. Black, tarry stools (melena) indicate upper GI bleeding (though may sometimes be caused by iron supplementation or bismuth). Bright red blood per rectum (haematochezia) suggests lower GI bleeding, often from the colon or rectum (e.g., haemorrhoids, IBD, infectious colitis). Pale, clay-coloured stools may indicate biliary obstruction.

4. Associated Symptoms:

Accompanying symptoms can further refine the differential diagnosis:

- Fever: Suggests an infectious etiology, particularly bacterial or parasitic. Fever is less common in viral gastroenteritis, but can occur. High fever is more typical of invasive bacterial infections.
- Abdominal Pain: Variable in diarrhea. Crampy abdominal pain is common in infectious gastroenteritis and IBS. Severe, localized abdominal pain may suggest inflammatory colitis or ischemic colitis. Pain relieved by defecation is often seen in IBS.

- Nausea and Vomiting: Frequently associated with viral gastroenteritis and food poisoning. Less prominent in colonic diarrhea.
- Weight Loss: Suggests chronic diarrhea and may point towards malabsorption syndromes (celiac disease, pancreatic insufficiency), IBD, or malignancy.
- Systemic Symptoms: Fatigue, malaise, joint pain, skin rashes, and eye inflammation may accompany IBD and some systemic infections.
- Dehydration: A serious complication of diarrhea, especially in young children, elderly individuals, and those with underlying comorbidities. Signs of dehydration include dry mucous membranes, decreased skin turgor, tachycardia, and hypotension.

Diagnostic Approaches:

The diagnostic approach to diarrhea should be tailored to the duration, severity, and associated features of the illness. A stepwise approach, starting with a thorough history and physical examination, followed by targeted investigations based on clinical suspicion, is generally recommended.

1. History and Physical Examination:

A detailed history is crucial. Key aspects to elicit include:

- Onset, duration, frequency, and volume of diarrhea.
- Stool characteristics: consistency, color, presence of blood, mucus, or fat.
- Associated symptoms: fever, abdominal pain, nausea, vomiting, weight loss, systemic symptoms.
- Travel history: Risk of traveller's diarrhea.
- Dietary history: Recent food intake (food poisoning), lactose intolerance, dietary changes.
- Medication history: Antibiotics (C. *difficile* infection), laxatives, NSAIDs, other medications known to cause diarrhea.

- Past medical history: History of IBD, celiac disease, IBS, diabetes, immunocompromised state.
- Family history: Family history of IBD, celiac disease, or colon cancer.

Physical examination should focus on:

- Hydration status: Assess mucous membranes, skin turgor, capillary refill, orthostatic vital signs.
- Abdominal examination: Auscultate bowel sounds, palpate for tenderness, masses, or organomegaly. Assess for signs of peritonitis if pain is severe.
- Rectal examination: Assess for haemorrhoids, fissures, and faecal impaction. Stool for occult blood testing can be obtained.
- General examination: Look for signs of systemic illness, such as fever, rash, jaundice, or lymphadenopathy.

2. Initial Investigations (Often for Acute Diarrhea):

For mild to moderate acute diarrhea in otherwise healthy adults, further investigations are often unnecessary, particularly if symptoms are suggestive of viral gastroenteritis and there are no alarm features (bloody diarrhea, severe dehydration, high fever, severe abdominal pain, immunocompromised status). Symptomatic treatment with oral rehydration solutions and dietary modifications is typically sufficient.

However, in cases of persistent diarrhea, severe symptoms, or presence of alarm features, initial investigations may include:

- Stool studies:
    - Stool microscopy for faecal leukocytes: Presence of leukocytes suggests inflammatory diarrhea, often bacterial or IBD. Absence does not rule out inflammatory causes but is more typical of viral or toxin-mediated diarrhea.

- Stool for ova and parasites (O&P): Indicated in cases of persistent diarrhea, travel history to endemic areas, or suspicion of parasitic infection (e.g., *Giardia, Entamoeba*).
- Stool bacterial culture: Recommended for bloody diarrhea, severe diarrhea, persistent diarrhea, fever, or immunocompromised patients, to identify bacterial pathogens like *Salmonella*, *Shigella*, *Campylobacter*, and EHEC.
- *Clostridium difficile* toxin assay: Perform in patients with recent antibiotic use, healthcare-associated diarrhea, or suspected pseudomembranous colitis. PCR or enzyme immunoassay are common methods.
- Stool for faecal calprotectin or lactoferrin: Inflammatory markers in stool, useful for differentiating inflammatory from non-inflammatory diarrhea, particularly in chronic diarrhea and suspected IBD or microscopic colitis.
- Stool fat quantification (72-hour faecal fat test or Sudan stain): Indicated for suspected fat malabsorption and steatorrhea (though less commonly performed now, often replaced by less cumbersome tests).

- Blood tests:
  - Complete blood count (CBC): May show leucocytosis in infectious or inflammatory diarrhea. Anemia may be present in chronic diarrhea or IBD.
  - Electrolytes (sodium, potassium, chloride, bicarbonate): Assess for electrolyte imbalances due to diarrhea, especially in severe or prolonged cases.
  - Renal function tests (BUN, creatinine): Evaluate hydration status and renal function, particularly in dehydrated patients.
  - C-reactive protein (CRP) or erythrocyte sedimentation rate (ESR): Elevated inflammatory markers may suggest IBD or inflammatory colitis, but are non-specific.

3. Advanced Investigations (Often for Chronic Diarrhea):

If initial investigations are unrevealing or if chronic diarrhea persists, further investigations are warranted to explore less common etiologies. These may include:

- Colonoscopy or sigmoidoscopy with biopsies: Essential for evaluating chronic diarrhea, bloody diarrhea, and suspected IBD, microscopic colitis, or malignancy. Allows for visualization of the colonic mucosa, detection of mucosal inflammation, ulceration, polyps, or tumors, and obtaining tissue biopsies for histological examination.
- Upper endoscopy with duodenal biopsies: Indicated for suspected malabsorption, celiac disease, or upper GI causes of diarrhea. Duodenal biopsies are crucial for diagnosing celiac disease.
- Small bowel imaging (CT enterography, MR enterography, capsule endoscopy): Used to evaluate Crohn's disease affecting the small bowel, small bowel tumors, or other small bowel pathologies when colonoscopy and upper endoscopy are non-diagnostic. Capsule endoscopy can be particularly useful for visualizing the small bowel mucosa.
- Abdominal CT scan: May be performed to evaluate for intra-abdominal abscesses, masses, or other structural abnormalities in patients with persistent diarrhea, abdominal pain, or suspected complications.
- Hydrogen breath tests: Used to diagnose lactose intolerance, fructose malabsorption, and small intestinal bacterial overgrowth (SIBO).
- Pancreatic function tests (faecal elastase-1, secretin stimulation test): Indicated for suspected pancreatic insufficiency, particularly in patients with steatorrhea, weight loss, or chronic diarrhea. faecal elastase-1 is a non-invasive screening test.
- Thyroid function tests: Rule out hyperthyroidism in patients with unexplained diarrhea and other suggestive symptoms.

- Serum markers for celiac disease (tissue transglutaminase IgA, endomysial antibody IgA): Screening tests for celiac disease, particularly in patients with chronic diarrhea, malabsorption, or family history of celiac disease.
- 24-hour stool collection for volume and electrolytes: May be helpful in differentiating osmotic from secretory diarrhea, particularly in refractory cases.
- Specific hormone levels (serum gastrin, vasoactive intestinal peptide (VIP), calcitonin, serotonin metabolites [5-HIAA]): Considered in rare cases of suspected endocrine tumors causing secretory diarrhea.

A Comparative Summary:

Diarrhoea Type	Key Presentations	Diagnostic Tests	Common Causes
Acute Diarrhoea	Sudden onset, usually lasting less than 2 weeks. May be watery, bloody, or mucoid depending on the cause. Often accompanied by nausea, vomiting, abdominal cramps, and fever.	Usually, clinical diagnosis based on history and physical exam. Stool culture may be indicated if symptoms are severe, persistent, bloody, or associated with fever. Sometimes, stool antigen tests for specific pathogens (e.g., *C. difficile*, Rotavirus) are used.	Infectious agents: Viruses (Norovirus, Rotavirus), Bacteria (*Salmonella*, *E.coli*, *Campylobacter*), Parasites (*Giardia*, *Cryptosporidium*). Food poisoning: Bacterial toxins. Medications: Antibiotics, certain laxatives. Traveler's diarrhoea.
Chronic Diarrhoea	Diarrhoea lasting for 4 weeks or more. Symptoms can be persistent or intermittent. May be associated with weight loss, fatigue, and nutritional deficiencies. Stool characteristics can vary widely.	More extensive investigation often required. Stool studies: Faecal calprotectin (for inflammation), stool culture, ova and parasites, *C. difficile* toxin. Blood tests: Complete blood count, electrolytes, inflammatory markers, thyroid function, coeliac serology. Endoscopy, Colonoscopy, upper endoscopy with biopsies. Imaging: CT scan or MRI of the abdomen/pelvis may be considered.	Irritable Bowel Syndrome (IBS). Inflammatory Bowel Disease (IBD): Crohn's disease, Ulcerative colitis, microscopic colitis. Coeliac disease. Malabsorption syndromes: Lactose intolerance, Pancreatic insufficiency, Bile acid malabsorption. Endocrine disorders: Hyperthyroidism, Diabetes. Chronic infections. Medications. Certain cancers.

Osmotic Diarrhoea	Large volume, watery diarrhoea. *Decreases or stops with fasting*. May be associated with bloating and gas. Stool osmolality gap is high.	Stool osmolality and electrolytes. Detailed dietary history looking for osmotically active substances. Lactose tolerance test, hydrogen breath test (for carbohydrate malabsorption). Assessment for laxative use.	Lactulose or magnesium-containing laxatives. Lactose intolerance. Ingestion of poorly absorbed carbohydrates: Artificial sweeteners (sorbitol, mannitol) found in sugar-free products. Malabsorption of nutrients.
Secretory Diarrhoea	Large volume, watery diarrhoea that *persists even with fasting*. May lead to dehydration and electrolyte imbalances. Stool osmolality gap is low.	Stool electrolytes. Assessment for medication use. Hormone assays (if endocrine cause suspected). Colonoscopy to rule out tumours.	Bacterial toxins: Cholera toxin, Enterotoxigenic *E. coli* (ETEC). Hormone-secreting tumours: VIPoma, Gastrinomas. Certain medications: Stimulant laxatives, some chemotherapy drugs. Bile acid malabsorption (sometimes classified as secretory).
Inflammatory Diarrhoea	Bloody or mucoid diarrhoea. Often associated with abdominal pain, fever, urgency, and tenesmus (feeling of incomplete evacuation). May be smaller volume compared to osmotic or secretory types.	Stool studies: Faecal leukocytes, lactoferrin, calprotectin, stool culture. Sigmoidoscopy or colonoscopy with biopsies is often crucial to visualize the intestinal mucosa and obtain tissue for microscopic examination.	Inflammatory Bowel Disease (IBD): Crohn's disease, Ulcerative colitis. Infectious colitis: *Shigella*, *Salmonella*, *Campylobacter*, *C. difficile* colitis. Ischaemic colitis. Radiation

Differential Diagnosis of malabsorption.

Introduction:

Malabsorption, a condition characterized by the impaired intestinal absorption of nutrients, stands as a significant clinical challenge across the globe. It is not a disease in itself, but rather a consequence of various underlying pathologies that disrupt the intricate processes of digestion and nutrient uptake within the gastrointestinal tract. The clinical spectrum of malabsorption is vast and varied, ranging from subtle nutrient deficiencies presenting with vague symptoms to severe, life-threatening conditions marked by profound weight loss, debilitating diarrhea, and systemic manifestations.

The consequences of malabsorption extend beyond mere nutritional deficiencies. They impact every organ system, affecting growth and development in children, reducing quality of life in adults, and contributing to increased morbidity and mortality across all age groups. Timely and accurate diagnosis is therefore paramount, not only to alleviate symptoms and prevent long-term complications, but also to identify and address the underlying cause, which may range from readily treatable infections to chronic inflammatory conditions, structural abnormalities, or even malignancies.

The journey to diagnosing malabsorption can be complex and often requires a systematic and meticulous approach. The diverse etiological landscape of malabsorption, coupled with the overlapping clinical presentations of its various causes, necessitates a robust understanding of the differential diagnosis. This chapter aims to provide a comprehensive and clinically relevant guide to the differential diagnosis of malabsorption. We will explore the key clinical presentations that should raise suspicion for malabsorption, delve into the diagnostic algorithms and investigations employed to unravel the underlying cause, present a comparative summary of the key differentiating features of major malabsorptive disorders, and finally, distill the essential takeaways for clinicians navigating this challenging area of gastroenterology. By integrating fundamental physiological principles with current diagnostic strategies and recent research advancements, this chapter strives to equip the reader with the knowledge and tools necessary to effectively approach the patient with suspected malabsorption and arrive at an accurate and timely diagnosis.

Understanding Malabsorption: A Foundation for Differential Diagnosis

To effectively navigate the differential diagnosis of malabsorption, it is crucial to first establish a solid foundation in the physiology of digestion and absorption, the pathophysiology of malabsorptive states, and a systematic classification of malabsorption disorders.

1. The Orchestrated Symphony of Digestion and Absorption: A Physiological Review

Normal digestion and absorption are complex, highly coordinated processes that occur throughout the gastrointestinal tract, transforming complex food components into absorbable molecules. This intricate symphony involves mechanical, chemical, and enzymatic breakdown of food, followed by the transport of nutrients across the intestinal mucosa into the bloodstream or lymphatic system. For the purpose of understanding malabsorption, it is helpful to consider the key stages and components of this intricate process.

- Luminal Digestion: The process begins in the mouth with mastication, which increases the surface area of food for enzymatic action. As food enters the stomach, gastric acid and pepsin initiate protein digestion. However, the bulk of luminal digestion occurs in the small intestine. Here, pancreatic enzymes (amylase for carbohydrates, lipase and colipase for fats, proteases like trypsin and chymotrypsin for proteins) and bile salts (secreted by the liver and stored in the gallbladder) play crucial roles.

  - Carbohydrate Digestion: Dietary carbohydrates, mainly polysaccharides and disaccharides, are hydrolyzed by salivary and pancreatic amylase into smaller oligosaccharides and disaccharides.
  - Protein Digestion: Proteins are broken down by gastric pepsin and pancreatic proteases into smaller peptides and amino acids.
  - Fat Digestion: Triglycerides are emulsified by bile salts, increasing their surface area for the action of pancreatic lipase. Lipase, aided by colipase, hydrolyzes triglycerides into monoglycerides and free fatty acids. Micelles, formed by bile salts, monoglycerides, and fatty acids, are essential for transporting fats to the intestinal brush border for absorption.

- Brush Border Digestion: The brush border of the enterocytes, the absorptive cells lining the small intestine, contains enzymes that further digest carbohydrates and peptides. Disaccharidases (lactase, sucrase-isomaltose, maltase) break down disaccharides into monosaccharides (glucose, fructose, galactose). Peptidases complete the digestion of small peptides into amino acids.
- Mucosal Absorption: Once digested into absorbable units, nutrients are transported across the enterocyte membrane. This process involves various mechanisms:

  - Monosaccharide Absorption: Glucose and galactose are absorbed via active transport, mediated by sodium-glucose cotransporter 1 (SGLT1). Fructose is absorbed by facilitated diffusion via GLUT5. All monosaccharides eventually exit the enterocyte via GLUT2 into the bloodstream.
  - Amino Acid Absorption: Amino acids are absorbed via several sodium-dependent and sodium-independent active transport systems.

- Fat Absorption: Monoglycerides and fatty acids, within micelles, diffuse across the enterocyte membrane. Inside the enterocyte, they are re-esterified into triglycerides, packaged with cholesterol and apolipoproteins into chylomicrons. Chylomicrons are transported into the lymphatic system, eventually reaching the systemic circulation. Short- and medium-chain fatty acids can be absorbed directly into the portal circulation.
- Vitamin and Mineral Absorption: Vitamins and minerals have specific absorption mechanisms, which can be complex and vary depending on the nutrient. For example, vitamin B12 absorption requires intrinsic factor secreted by parietal cells in the stomach and specific receptors in the terminal ileum. Fat-soluble vitamins (A, D, E, K) are absorbed with fats and require bile salts for solubilization. Minerals like iron and calcium also have specialized transport systems, often regulated by the body's nutritional status.

- Water and Electrolyte Absorption: The small intestine absorbs a significant amount of water and electrolytes. Sodium, chloride, and water absorption are tightly coupled. The colon primarily absorbs water and electrolytes, further concentrating faecal contents.

2. Pathophysiology of Malabsorption: Disruptions in the Digestive Symphony

Malabsorption arises when one or more of these intricate steps in digestion and absorption are disrupted. The underlying mechanisms can be broadly categorized into:

- Defective Luminal Digestion: This occurs when there is insufficient breakdown of food in the intestinal lumen. Common causes include:
  - Pancreatic Exocrine Insufficiency (PEI): Lack of pancreatic enzymes due to conditions like chronic pancreatitis, cystic

fibrosis, pancreatic cancer, or pancreatic surgery impairs the digestion of fats, proteins, and carbohydrates. Fat malabsorption is particularly prominent in PEI due to the crucial role of pancreatic lipase.

- Bile Salt Deficiency: Inadequate bile salt production (e.g., liver disease) or impaired delivery to the intestinal lumen (e.g., bile duct obstruction, ileal resection) leads to impaired fat emulsification and micelle formation, resulting in fat malabsorption.
- Gastric Hyperacidity: While gastric acid is essential for initial protein digestion, excessive acid production (e.g., Zollinger-Ellison syndrome) can inactivate pancreatic lipase and precipitate bile salts in the jejunum, contributing to fat malabsorption. Conversely, gastric hypoacidity (e.g., atrophic gastritis, proton pump inhibitor use) can impair protein digestion and vitamin B12 absorption by affecting intrinsic factor binding.

- Defective Brush Border Digestion: Enzyme deficiencies at the brush border impair the final stages of digestion. The most common example is:
  - Lactase Deficiency: Congenital or acquired deficiency of lactase, the enzyme that breaks down lactose into glucose and galactose, leads to lactose malabsorption, causing symptoms like bloating, gas, and diarrhea upon lactose ingestion.
  - Sucrase-Isomaltose Deficiency: Less common, but can cause similar symptoms after sucrose intake.

- Defective Mucosal Absorption: This is the most common category and involves damage to the intestinal mucosa, leading to impaired nutrient uptake. Causes include:
  - Small Intestinal Mucosal Diseases: Conditions like celiac disease, Crohn's disease, microscopic colitis, infectious

enteritis (e.g., giardiasis, cryptosporidiosis), tropical sprue, and radiation enteritis damage the intestinal villi, reduce the absorptive surface area, and impair enterocyte function.

- Short Bowel Syndrome (SBS): Surgical resection or congenital absence of a significant portion of the small intestine reduces the absorptive capacity, leading to malabsorption, particularly if the ileum is involved, which is the primary site for bile salt and vitamin B12 absorption.
- Lymphatic Obstruction: Conditions that block intestinal lymphatics (e.g., intestinal lymphangiectasia, lymphoma) impair the transport of chylomicrons and fat-soluble vitamins, leading to fat malabsorption and protein-losing enteropathy.
- Vascular Insufficiency: Ischemic bowel disease can damage the intestinal mucosa and impair absorption.

- Post-Absorptive Factors: Less commonly, malabsorption can be due to factors beyond the intestinal mucosa, such as:
    - Abnormal Intestinal Permeability: Increased intestinal permeability ("leaky gut") can lead to nutrient loss and inflammation.
    - Impaired Nutrient Transport: Rare genetic disorders can affect specific nutrient transporters, leading to selective malabsorption (e.g., glucose-galactose malabsorption, congenital folate malabsorption).
    - Systemic Diseases: Certain systemic diseases can indirectly cause malabsorption, such as hyperthyroidism (increased intestinal motility), diabetes mellitus (autonomic neuropathy affecting gut motility and secretion), and certain medications.

3. Classification of Malabsorption: Structuring the Differential

To effectively approach the differential diagnosis, it is helpful to classify malabsorption disorders based on different criteria. Common classifications include:

- Global vs. Selective Malabsorption:
  - Global Malabsorption (Generalized): Indicates malabsorption of multiple nutrients, typically due to widespread mucosal damage or extensive intestinal resection. Examples: celiac disease, severe Crohn's disease, short bowel syndrome.
  - Selective Malabsorption (Specific Nutrient): Malabsorption of a single nutrient or a limited group of nutrients, often due to specific enzyme deficiencies, transporter defects, or localized lesions. Examples: lactase deficiency (carbohydrate), vitamin B12 malabsorption (vitamin), iron deficiency anaemia (iron).

- Based on Underlying Mechanism (as discussed above):
  - Luminal Digestion Defects
  - Brush Border Digestion Defects
  - Mucosal Absorption Defects
  - Post-Absorptive Defects

- Based on Anatomical Location of Defect:
  - Gastric Malabsorption: Primarily affects iron, vitamin B12, and calcium absorption due to altered pH, intrinsic factor deficiency, and rapid transit.
  - Small Intestinal Malabsorption: Affects a wide range of nutrients, including carbohydrates, fats, proteins, vitamins, and minerals. The site within the small intestine (duodenum, jejunum, ileum) can further refine the differential (e.g., duodenum – iron, folate, calcium; jejunum – carbohydrates, proteins, fats; ileum – bile salts, vitamin B12).
  - Colonic Malabsorption: Primarily involved in water and electrolyte malabsorption. Insignificant for macronutrient malabsorption under normal circumstances.

This classification framework provides a structured approach to considering the potential causes of malabsorption based on the clinical presentation, laboratory findings, and imaging studies. It helps to narrow down the differential diagnosis and guide further investigations.

Key Presentations of Malabsorption: Recognizing the Clinical Clues

The clinical manifestations of malabsorption are incredibly diverse, reflecting the wide range of nutrients that can be affected and the variable severity of the underlying condition. Symptoms can be broad categorized into gastrointestinal (GI) manifestations and systemic manifestations arising from nutrient deficiencies.

1. Gastrointestinal Manifestations: The Gut's Cry for Help

GI symptoms are often the most prominent and earliest indicators of malabsorption, prompting patients to seek medical attention. However, they are often non-specific and can overlap with symptoms of other gastrointestinal disorders. A detailed history and careful evaluation of these symptoms are crucial.

- Diarrhea: The hallmark GI symptom of malabsorption. Diarrhea can be characterized by increased stool frequency, increased stool volume, and altered stool consistency. Different types of diarrhea are associated with different types of malabsorption:

    - Steatorrhea (Fatty Diarrhea): Bulky, pale, foul-smelling stools that float or stick to the toilet bowl. Indicates fat malabsorption due to pancreatic insufficiency, bile salt deficiency, or small intestinal disease. May be accompanied by oily droplets in the stool or faecal incontinence.
    - Watery Diarrhea: Large volume, watery stools, often associated with carbohydrate malabsorption (e.g., lactose intolerance) or secretory diarrhea (some infections, inflammatory bowel disease).
    - Small Volume, Frequent Diarrhea: May occur in inflammatory conditions like Crohn's disease or microscopic colitis, often associated with urgency and tenesmus.

- Abdominal Pain and Discomfort: Abdominal pain can be variable, ranging from mild discomfort and bloating to severe cramping pain.
    - Cramping Pain: Often associated with gas and bloating, particularly after meals, may suggest carbohydrate malabsorption (e.g., lactose intolerance) or small intestinal bacterial overgrowth (SIBO).
    - Diffuse Abdominal Pain: May be seen in inflammatory bowel disease, celiac disease, or chronic pancreatitis.
- Bloating and Distension: Excessive gas production and fluid accumulation in the intestines can lead to abdominal bloating and distension. Common in carbohydrate malabsorption, SIBO, and conditions affecting intestinal motility.
- Increased Flatus: Excessive gas production, often foul-smelling, is another symptom of carbohydrate malabsorption and SIBO.
- Weight Loss: Unintentional weight loss is a significant indicator of malabsorption, particularly when it is progressive and unexplained by dietary changes or increased physical activity. The degree of weight loss can range from mild to severe and depends on the severity and duration of malabsorption.
- Nausea and Vomiting: May occur in some conditions causing malabsorption, such as celiac disease, Crohn's disease, or gastroparesis (which can indirectly affect nutrient absorption).
- Anorexia (Loss of Appetite): Can be a symptom of underlying inflammatory conditions or systemic illness contributing to malabsorption.

Differential Diagnosis of Dysphagia

Introduction: The Multifaceted Nature of Swallowing Difficulties

Dysphagia, or difficulty swallowing, is a prevalent clinical problem affecting individuals across the lifespan, from neonates to the elderly. It is not a disease itself, but rather a symptom of an underlying medical condition disrupting the intricate and coordinated process of transporting food and liquids from the mouth to the stomach. The implications of dysphagia extend far beyond mere inconvenience. It can lead to serious health consequences, including malnutrition, dehydration, aspiration pneumonia, airway obstruction, and even death. Furthermore, dysphagia significantly impacts quality of life, affecting social participation, emotional well-being, and overall functional independence.

Given the diverse and often overlapping presentations of dysphagia, a systematic approach to differential diagnosis is paramount. Accurate and timely identification of the underlying etiology is crucial to guide appropriate management strategies, minimize complications, and improve patient outcomes. This chapter will delve into the complexities of dysphagia differential diagnosis, exploring key clinical presentations, outlining essential diagnostic approaches, providing a comparative summary of common dysphagic conditions, and highlighting key takeaways for clinicians. By understanding the nuances of dysphagia and adopting a methodical diagnostic framework, healthcare professionals can effectively navigate the diagnostic challenges and provide optimal care for individuals experiencing swallowing difficulties.

Key Presentations: Deciphering the Symptom Spectrum of Dysphagia

Dysphagia manifests through a wide array of signs and symptoms, varying in severity and nature depending on the location and underlying cause of the swallowing impairment. While patients may broadly report "difficulty swallowing," a detailed exploration of their specific symptoms is crucial for narrowing the differential diagnosis. Symptoms can be broadly categorized based on the phase of swallowing affected (oral, pharyngeal, oesophageal) and by the type of bolus (liquids, solids, or both).

1. Oral Phase Dysphagia: Difficulties at this stage arise from impaired oral control and manipulation of food. Key presentations include:

- Difficulty Chewing: Prolonged chewing time, inability to masticate solid foods effectively, fatigue during chewing. Suggests issues with dentition, oral motor strength, or sensory awareness.
- Oral Leakage/Drooling: Food or liquid escaping from the mouth before or during the swallow. Indicates poor lip closure, reduced tongue control, or impaired oral containment.
- Food Pocketing: Food residue remaining in the cheeks, sulci, or under the tongue after swallowing. Reflects reduced oral sensation, decreased tongue strength and coordination, or impaired buccal muscle function.
- Slow Oral Transit: Prolonged time to move the bolus from the front to the back of the mouth. Points to reduced tongue movement speed, strength, or coordination.
- Difficulty Initiating Swallow: Hesitation or reluctance to swallow, multiple attempts to initiate a swallow. May indicate sensory processing difficulties, apraxia of swallow, or neurological deficits impacting the swallow trigger.

2. Pharyngeal Phase Dysphagia: Difficulties in this phase involve the rapid and complex sequence of events that propel the bolus through the pharynx and protect the airway. Key presentations are often more alarming and carry higher risks:

- Coughing or Choking During or Immediately After Swallowing: Reflects aspiration (bolus entering the airway) or penetration (bolus entering the larynx but not below the vocal cords). Indicates impaired airway protection mechanisms, reduced pharyngeal peristalsis, or delayed swallow response.
- Wet or Gurgle Voice After Swallowing: Suggests pooling of secretions or food residue in the pharynx or larynx after the swallow, often due to pharyngeal weakness or reduced laryngeal elevation.
- Nasal Regurgitation: Food or liquid entering the nasal cavity during swallowing. Indicates velopharyngeal insufficiency,

preventing the closure of the nasopharynx during the pharyngeal phase.

- Multiple Swallows per Bolus: Needing to swallow repeatedly to clear food from the pharynx. Suggests inefficient pharyngeal clearance, reduced peristaltic strength, or pharyngeal residue.
- Globus Sensation: A persistent feeling of a lump or foreign body in the throat, even when swallowing is not occurring. While often psychogenic, it can also be associated with pharyngeal muscle tension or reflux.

3. Esophageal Phase Dysphagia: Difficulties in this phase relate to the transport of the bolus through the esophagus into the stomach. Patients often describe a sensation of food sticking in their chest or throat:

- Sensation of Food Sticking in the Throat or Chest: Patients can often pinpoint the location of obstruction, which can help differentiate between oropharyngeal and esophageal dysphagia.
- Chest Pain During or After Swallowing: May suggest esophageal spasm, esophagitis, or other esophageal motility disorders.
- Heartburn or Acid Reflux: Symptoms of gastroesophageal reflux disease (GERD), which can contribute to esophageal dysphagia.
- Regurgitation of Undigested Food: Food returning from the esophagus, often hours after eating, suggests esophageal obstruction or motility problems like achalasia.
- Weight Loss and Malnutrition: In severe cases, esophageal dysphagia can lead to reduced oral intake and subsequent nutritional deficiencies.

4. Specific Bolus Consistency Difficulties: The type of bolus that provokes dysphagia can provide clues to the underlying etiology.

- Dysphagia Primarily for Liquids: Suggests potential weakness or incoordination in the oropharyngeal phase, particularly in the timing and coordination required to manage thin liquids.

Neurological conditions and pharyngeal weakness are often implicated.

- Dysphagia Primarily for Solids: May point towards structural obstructions in the esophagus, such as strictures, tumors, or esophageal webs. Motility disorders or sensory deficits can also contribute.
- Dysphagia for Both Liquids and Solids: Indicates a more generalized swallowing impairment, possibly encompassing both oropharyngeal and esophageal phases. Neuromuscular disorders, diffuse motility disorders, or advanced structural lesions should be considered.

Differential Diagnosis: A Framework for Identifying the Root Cause

Dysphagia is a symptom with a vast differential diagnosis. To effectively navigate this complexity, it is helpful to categorize potential etiologies into broad groups. This section will explore major categories of conditions that can cause dysphagia, highlighting key characteristics and differentiating features.

1. Neurological Dysphagia: Neurological disorders are a leading cause of dysphagia, as they disrupt the complex neural control of swallowing.

- Stroke (Cerebrovascular Accident - CVA): Stroke is a common cause of dysphagia, particularly in the acute phase. Dysphagia can result from damage to cortical swallowing centers, brainstem nuclei, or corticobulbar tracts. Presentations vary depending on the stroke location and severity, but often involve both oral and pharyngeal phase deficits, including weakness, incoordination, sensory loss, and impaired swallow reflex.
    - Key Presentations: Unilateral weakness, hemiparesis, aphasia, neglect, sensory deficits, oral and pharyngeal phase dysphagia, aspiration risk, variable recovery.
    - Differentiating Features: Sudden onset, focal neurological deficits consistent with vascular territory, neuroimaging confirmation (CT or MRI).

- Parkinson's Disease (PD): Progressive neurodegenerative disorder affecting dopamine-producing neurons. Dysphagia in PD is related to motor deficits, rigidity, bradykinesia, and postural instability impacting all phases of swallowing.
  - Key Presentations: Tremor, rigidity, bradykinesia, postural instability, drooling, prolonged oral transit, pharyngeal residue, esophageal dysmotility (often affecting peristalsis). Progresses over time.
  - Differentiating Features: Classic Parkinsonian motor symptoms, response to dopaminergic medications, slow and progressive onset.

- Multiple Sclerosis (MS): Autoimmune disease affecting the central nervous system myelin. Dysphagia in MS can result from lesions in various locations within the brain and spinal cord, leading to diverse swallowing impairments.
  - Key Presentations: Variable and fluctuating symptoms depending on lesion location and disease course. Can involve oral, pharyngeal, and esophageal dysphagia, often with spasticity, fatigue, and sensory deficits.
  - Differentiating Features: Relapsing-remitting or progressive neurological symptoms, optic neuritis, fatigue, sensory disturbances, characteristic MRI findings of white matter lesions.

- Amyotrophic Lateral Sclerosis (ALS): Progressive neurodegenerative disease affecting motor neurons. Dysphagia in ALS is a significant and debilitating symptom, resulting from progressive weakness of bulbar muscles (tongue, pharynx, larynx).
  - Key Presentations: Progressive muscle weakness, fasciculations, bulbar symptoms (dysarthria, dysphagia, dyspnea), both upper and lower motor neuron signs, initially

oral phase difficulties progressing to severe oropharyngeal dysphagia and aspiration.
  - Differentiating Features: Progressive and relentless course, muscle atrophy and fasciculations, both upper and lower motor neuron signs, EMG findings.

- Myasthenia Gravis (MG): Autoimmune neuromuscular junction disorder causing muscle weakness that worsens with activity and improves with rest. Dysphagia in MG is due to muscle weakness affecting the oropharyngeal and esophageal muscles.
  - Key Presentations: Fatigable weakness, ptosis, diplopia, dysarthria, dysphagia that worsens with prolonged swallowing attempts or repeated meals, nasal regurgitation, improved strength after rest or with anticholinesterase medications.
  - Differentiating Features: Fluctuating weakness, fatigability, positive acetylcholine receptor antibodies, improvement with anticholinesterase medication (Tensilon test), EMG findings of neuromuscular junction defect.

- Brain Tumors: Tumors in the brainstem, cranial nerves, or surrounding structures can directly compress or disrupt neural pathways involved in swallowing.
  - Key Presentations: Progressive neurological deficits depending on tumor location, headaches, nausea, vomiting, seizures, cranial nerve palsies, dysphagia may be gradual or sudden onset depending on tumor growth rate and location.
  - Differentiating Features: Progressive neurological deficits, imaging evidence of brain tumor (CT or MRI), focal neurological signs.

- Traumatic Brain Injury (TBI): Head trauma can cause diffuse or focal neurological damage, leading to dysphagia. Severity and type of dysphagia depend on the extent and location of injury.

- Key Presentations: Variable depending on injury severity and location, ranging from mild oral phase difficulties to severe oropharyngeal dysphagia with aspiration risk, cognitive impairments may complicate diagnosis and management.
- Differentiating Features: History of head trauma, neurological deficits, imaging evidence of brain injury (CT or MRI).

- Dementia: Cognitive decline in dementia can indirectly impact swallowing function. Reduced attention, impaired sequencing, and decreased self-awareness can lead to unsafe eating habits and dysphagia.
    - Key Presentations: Progressive cognitive decline, memory loss, judgment and reasoning impairment, swallowing difficulties often emerge later in the disease course, oral phase difficulties, food pocketing, slow eating rate, decreased self-feeding skills.
    - Differentiating Features: Progressive cognitive decline, memory impairment, behavioral changes, neuropsychological testing findings.

2. Structural/Mechanical Dysphagia: Physical obstructions or anatomical abnormalities in the swallowing pathway can impede bolus transit.

- Esophageal Strictures: Narrowing of the esophageal lumen, often caused by chronic GERD, peptic ulcer disease, caustic ingestion, radiation therapy, or esophageal surgery.
    - Key Presentations: Solid food dysphagia that is progressive, heartburn, regurgitation, history of GERD or risk factors for stricture formation.
    - Differentiating Features: Progressive dysphagia for solids, history of GERD or risk factors, EGD visualization of stricture and biopsy, barium swallow showing narrowing.

- Esophageal Tumors (Benign or Malignant): Growths within the esophageal lumen that can cause obstruction. Malignant tumors are a serious concern.
    - Key Presentations: Progressive dysphagia initially for solids then liquids, weight loss, odynophagia (painful swallowing), chest pain, hoarseness (if tumor involves recurrent laryngeal nerve), anemia, risk factors for esophageal cancer (smoking, alcohol, Barrett's esophagus).
    - Differentiating Features: Progressive dysphagia, weight loss, risk factors for esophageal cancer, EGD with biopsy confirming tumor, CT/PET scans for staging.

- Esophageal Webs and Rings (Schatzki Ring): Thin, web-like constrictions of the esophageal mucosa, often in the upper (webs) or lower (rings) esophagus. Schatzki ring is typically at the squamocolumnar junction.
    - Key Presentations: Intermittent solid food dysphagia, often described as "steakhouse dysphagia" when a large bolus gets stuck, may resolve spontaneously or with maneuvers like drinking liquids, often asymptomatic until a large bolus is ingested.
    - Differentiating Features: Intermittent dysphagia for solids, barium swallow demonstrating web or ring, EGD for visualization and dilation if needed.

- Esophageal Diverticula (Zenker's Diverticulum, Traction/Pulsion Diverticula): Outpouchings of the esophageal wall. Zenker's diverticulum is in the upper esophagus, while traction/pulsion diverticula are more distal.
    - Key Presentations (Zenker's): Regurgitation of undigested food and pills often hours after eating, halitosis, gurgling in the neck, feeling of a lump in the throat, aspiration risk due to retained food in the diverticulum.

- Key Presentations (Traction/Pulsion): Often asymptomatic, may cause dysphagia if large or cause motility disturbances.
- Differentiating Features (Zenker's): Regurgitation of undigested food, halitosis, barium swallow or esophagogram demonstrating diverticulum in the cervical esophagus. EGD should be performed cautiously to avoid perforation.
- Differentiating Features (Traction/Pulsion): Barium swallow or esophagogram demonstrating diverticulum, EGD to rule out other causes.

- Extrinsic Compression: External structures pressing on the esophagus, such as enlarged thyroid gland (goitre), mediastinal masses, cervical osteophytes, or vascular anomalies.

  - Key Presentations: Dysphagia that may be positional (worse in certain positions), gradual onset, depending on the nature and growth rate of the compressing structure.
  - Differentiating Features: Physical exam findings (goiter), imaging studies (CT, MRI) demonstrating extrinsic compression, history of relevant conditions.

3. Motility Disorders (Functional Dysphagia): Abnormalities in esophageal muscle contraction and coordination, without structural obstruction.

- Achalasia: Degeneration of esophageal neurons leading to impaired lower esophageal sphincter (LES) relaxation and esophageal aperistalsis.

  - Key Presentations: Progressive dysphagia for both solids and liquids, regurgitation of undigested food (often nocturnal), chest pain, weight loss, slow eating, "bird's beak" appearance on barium swallow (dilated esophagus, narrowed distal segment).
  - Differentiating Features: Dysphagia for both solids and liquids, regurgitation, barium swallow findings, esophageal

manometry showing absent peristalsis and incomplete LES relaxation.

- Diffuse Esophageal Spasm (DES): Uncoordinated and often painful esophageal contractions.
    - Key Presentations: Intermittent chest pain (angina-like), dysphagia for both solids and liquids, "corkscrew esophagus" appearance on barium swallow (multiple simultaneous contractions). Manometry is key for diagnosis.
    - Differentiating Features: Intermittent chest pain, dysphagia, barium swallow findings, esophageal manometry demonstrating simultaneous contractions.
- Nutcracker Esophagus (Hypercontractile Esophagus): Abnormally forceful esophageal contractions, often associated with reflux.
    - Key Presentations: Chest pain, dysphagia (less prominent than in DES or achalasia), often associated with GERD symptoms. Manometry is diagnostic showing high-amplitude peristaltic contractions

Differential Diagnosis of Hepatomegaly

Introduction

Hepatomegaly, the enlargement of the liver, is a frequently encountered clinical finding, palpable during routine abdominal examinations or incidentally detected through imaging studies. It serves as a critical indicator of underlying pathology, signalling a wide spectrum of diseases ranging from benign conditions to life-threatening illnesses. Understanding the differential diagnosis of hepatomegaly is paramount for clinicians across various specialties, as timely and accurate diagnosis significantly impacts patient management and prognosis. This chapter aims to provide a comprehensive guide to navigating the complex landscape of hepatomegaly, encompassing key clinical presentations, structured diagnostic approaches, a comparative summary of diverse etiologies, and essential takeaways for clinical practice.

Key Presentations of Hepatomegaly

The clinical presentation of hepatomegaly is highly variable, influenced by the underlying etiology, the rate of liver enlargement, and the presence of associated complications. Hepatomegaly can be broadly classified based on symptomatology:

1. Asymptomatic Hepatomegaly:

In many cases, hepatomegaly is discovered incidentally in asymptomatic individuals during routine physical examinations or imaging studies performed for unrelated reasons. This is particularly true in early stages of liver disease or in conditions that cause gradual liver enlargement. Asymptomatic hepatomegaly may be the sole presenting sign in:

- Early Non-Alcoholic Fatty Liver Disease (NAFLD): Mild to moderate hepatomegaly is a common finding in NAFLD, often without accompanying symptoms, especially in the early stages of steatosis.
- Compensated Chronic Liver Disease: In some patients with compensated cirrhosis, liver enlargement may be present without overt signs of decompensation like jaundice or ascites.
- Certain Storage Diseases: Conditions like glycogen storage diseases or mild haemochromatosis may initially present with asymptomatic hepatomegaly.
- Early Stages of Myeloproliferative Disorders: Splenomegaly is more classic, but hepatomegaly might be present in early myelofibrosis or polycythaemia vera.

In asymptomatic cases, carefully eliciting a detailed history and performing further investigations are crucial to unveil the underlying cause and prevent disease progression.

2. Symptomatic Hepatomegaly:

Symptomatic hepatomegaly manifests with a variety of clinical features, often reflecting the specific pathology affecting the liver. The symptoms can be categorized as follows:

- Right Upper Quadrant (RUQ) Pain or Discomfort: Liver enlargement can cause stretching of the Glisson's capsule, the fibrous covering of the liver, resulting in pain or a sensation of fullness in the RUQ. The nature of pain can vary:
    - Dull, aching pain: Often associated with slow, progressive liver enlargement, as seen in chronic liver disease, NAFLD, or congestive hepatomegaly.
    - Sharp, pleuritic pain: May indicate acute liver inflammation, such as acute hepatitis, or hepatic abscess.
    - Sudden, severe pain: Consider hepatic infarction, Budd-Chiari syndrome (acute hepatic venous outflow obstruction), or rupture of a hepatic tumor.
- Jaundice (Icterus): Yellowish discoloration of the skin and sclera due to hyperbilirubinemia. Jaundice in the context of hepatomegaly suggests hepatocellular dysfunction or biliary obstruction.
    - Hepatocellular Jaundice: Caused by impaired bilirubin conjugation or excretion by hepatocytes, seen in viral hepatitis, alcoholic hepatitis, drug-induced liver injury, and advanced cirrhosis.
    - Obstructive Jaundice: Results from blockage of bile flow, either intrahepatic (primary biliary cholangitis, primary sclerosing cholangitis, intrahepatic cholestasis of pregnancy) or extrahepatic (choledocholithiasis, cholangiocarcinoma, pancreatic cancer compressing the bile duct).

- Ascites and Peripheral Edema: Fluid accumulation in the peritoneal cavity (ascites) and peripheral tissues (edema) are common manifestations of portal hypertension and hypoalbuminemia, often seen in advanced chronic liver disease, cirrhosis, and congestive heart failure. Hepatomegaly in these cases is often accompanied by other signs of chronic liver disease, such as spider angiomata, palmar erythema, and muscle wasting.
- Gastrointestinal Symptoms: Nausea, vomiting, anorexia, and early satiety can occur due to liver enlargement and associated gastrointestinal dysmotility, or as systemic symptoms of underlying diseases like infections or malignancy.
- Systemic Symptoms: Fatigue, malaise, weight loss, fever, and night sweats may accompany hepatomegaly, particularly in infectious, inflammatory, or neoplastic conditions. Fever is prominent in acute infections (viral hepatitis, hepatic abscess, pyogenic cholangitis), while weight loss and night sweats raise suspicion for malignancy or chronic infections like tuberculosis.
- Bleeding Diathesis: Impaired liver synthesis of coagulation factors can lead to easy bruising, petechiae, and prolonged bleeding. This is more common in advanced liver disease and liver failure.
- Hepatic Encephalopathy: Altered mental status, confusion, and asterixis (liver flap) are signs of hepatic encephalopathy, a serious complication of liver failure. Hepatomegaly may be present or absent in these cases, as liver size can decrease in end-stage cirrhosis.

Diagnostic Approaches to Hepatomegaly

A systematic approach to diagnosing the cause of hepatomegaly is crucial. This involves a combination of history taking, physical examination, laboratory investigations, imaging studies, and liver biopsy in selected cases.

1. History and Physical Examination:

- Detailed History:
    - Medical History: Inquire about pre-existing liver disease, viral hepatitis risk factors (blood transfusions, intravenous drug use, unprotected sexual contact), alcohol consumption, medication history (prescription, over-the-counter, herbal supplements), travel history (endemic areas for parasitic infections), family history of liver disease, autoimmune disorders, metabolic diseases, and heart failure.
    - Symptom Onset and Duration: Acute onset suggests infection, drug-induced liver injury, or vascular events. Chronic onset points towards chronic liver diseases, metabolic disorders, or infiltrative processes.
    - Associated Symptoms: Carefully document the presence and nature of pain, jaundice, ascites, edema, gastrointestinal symptoms, systemic symptoms, and bleeding tendencies.
    - Occupational and Environmental Exposures: Exposure to hepatotoxic substances, toxins, or carcinogens.

- Physical Examination:
    - Liver Palpation: Assess liver size, consistency (firm, nodular, tender), and surface (smooth or irregular). Hepatomegaly is generally defined as liver span greater than 12 cm in the midclavicular line. Right costal margin palpation and percussion are crucial.
    - Signs of Chronic Liver Disease: Look for jaundice, spider angiomata, palmar erythema, gynecomastia, testicular atrophy, ascites, peripheral edema, muscle wasting, and asterixis.
    - Other Systemic Examination: Assess for lymphadenopathy (lymphoma, metastases, infections), splenomegaly (portal hypertension, hematological disorders, infections), cardiac

murmurs (congestive heart failure), and signs of underlying systemic diseases.

2. Laboratory Investigations:

- Liver Function Tests (LFTs): A cornerstone in the evaluation of hepatomegaly.
    - Aspartate Aminotransferase (AST) and Alanine Aminotransferase (ALT): Elevated in hepatocellular injury. Markedly elevated levels (>10 times upper limit of normal) suggest acute hepatitis (viral, alcoholic, drug-induced, autoimmune), ischemic hepatitis, or acute biliary obstruction. Mild to moderate elevations are seen in chronic hepatitis, NAFLD, and cirrhosis.
    - Alkaline Phosphatase (ALP) and Gamma-Glutamyl Transferase (GGT): Elevated in cholestatic liver disease (biliary obstruction, primary biliary cholangitis, primary sclerosing cholangitis). Isolated ALP elevation can also be seen in bone diseases. GGT confirms hepatic origin of elevated ALP.
    - Bilirubin (Total and Direct): Elevated in both hepatocellular and cholestatic jaundice. Direct bilirubin elevation is more specific for biliary obstruction or impaired bilirubin excretion.
    - Albumin: Reduced in chronic liver disease due to impaired synthetic function.
    - Prothrombin Time (PT) and International Normalized Ratio (INR): Prolonged in liver dysfunction due to decreased synthesis of coagulation factors.
    - Complete Blood Count (CBC): Assess for anaemia (chronic liver disease, bleeding, haemolysis), thrombocytopenia (portal hypertension, hypersplenism, bone marrow suppression), and leucocytosis (infection, inflammation, malignancy).
    - Renal Function Tests (BUN, Creatinine): Assess for hepatorenal syndrome in advanced liver disease or renal involvement in systemic diseases.

    - Electrolytes: Evaluate for electrolyte imbalances, especially hyponatremia in cirrhosis.

- Specific Serological and Molecular Tests: Targeted based on clinical suspicion.

    - Viral Hepatitis Serology: Hepatitis A, B, and C serologies are crucial to rule out viral hepatitis as a cause.
    - Autoimmune Markers: Antinuclear antibodies (ANA), anti-smooth muscle antibodies (ASMA), anti-liver kidney microsomal antibodies (anti-LKM1), anti-mitochondrial antibodies (AMA) are important for diagnosing autoimmune hepatitis and primary biliary cholangitis.
    - Iron Studies: Serum ferritin, transferrin saturation, and genetic testing for haemochromatosis (HFE gene mutations) if iron overload is suspected.
    - Alpha-1 Antitrypsin Level: Low levels suggest alpha-1 antitrypsin deficiency, a genetic cause of liver disease.
    - Ceruloplasmin and 24-hour Urine Copper: For Wilson's disease, especially in younger patients with liver disease or neurological symptoms.
    - Immunoglobulin Levels (IgG, IgM, IgA): Elevated IgG in autoimmune hepatitis, elevated IgM in primary biliary cholangitis.
    - Tumor Markers: Alpha-fetoprotein (AFP) for hepatocellular carcinoma (HCC), CA 19-9 for cholangiocarcinoma.
    - Blood Cultures: If infection is suspected, especially in febrile patients.
    - Specific Tests for Storage Diseases: Enzyme assays or genetic testing for glycogen storage diseases, lysosomal storage diseases (Gaucher disease, Niemann-Pick disease).

3. Imaging Studies:

- Ultrasound (USG) Abdomen: Often the initial imaging modality of choice.

- Advantages: Non-invasive, readily available, relatively inexpensive, no radiation, can assess liver size, echotexture (fatty liver, cirrhosis, masses), biliary dilatation, portal vein, hepatic veins, and presence of ascites. Doppler ultrasound can assess hepatic blood flow and patency of vessels (Budd-Chiari syndrome, portal vein thrombosis).
- Limitations: Operator-dependent, limited visualization in obese patients or with bowel gas interference, less sensitive for small lesions or subtle infiltrative diseases.

- Computed Tomography (CT) Scan Abdomen: Provides detailed anatomical information.
    - Advantages: Superior resolution for masses, abscesses, vascular abnormalities, and extrahepatic structures (pancreas, gallbladder, bile ducts). Can be performed with intravenous contrast to enhance vascular structures and characterize lesions.
    - Limitations: Radiation exposure, intravenous contrast allergy or nephrotoxicity risk, less sensitive for diffuse liver disease compared to ultrasound.

- Magnetic Resonance Imaging (MRI) Abdomen: Offers excellent soft tissue contrast and characterization of liver lesions.
    - Advantages: Superior for characterizing focal liver lesions (haemangiomas, adenomas, HCC, metastases), differentiating benign from malignant lesions, detecting iron overload and fatty infiltration, visualizing biliary tree (MRCP). No radiation exposure.
    - Limitations: More expensive, longer examination time, contraindicated in patients with certain metallic implants, motion artifacts, less readily available than ultrasound or CT.

- Liver Elastography (Fibro Scan or Shear Wave Elastography): Non-invasive assessment of liver stiffness, highly correlated with liver fibrosis stage. Useful in chronic liver diseases (NAFLD, viral hepatitis, alcoholic liver disease) to assess fibrosis progression and prognosis.
- Radioisotope Liver Scanning (Hepatobiliary Scintigraphy - HIDA Scan): Evaluates bile flow and biliary obstruction. Useful in suspected biliary atresia, choledochal cysts, and to assess gallbladder function.
- Angiography (Hepatic Venography, Portal Venography): Invasive procedure, less frequently used now due to non-invasive imaging. May be indicated in Budd-Chiari syndrome or portal hypertension evaluation, especially when interventional procedures (TIPS, balloon angioplasty) are considered.

4. Liver Biopsy:

Liver biopsy is the gold standard for definitive diagnosis in many cases of hepatomegaly, especially when non-invasive methods are inconclusive or when histological information is critical for diagnosis, prognosis, and treatment planning.

- Indications for Liver Biopsy in Hepatomegaly:
    - Undiagnosed hepatomegaly after non-invasive investigations.
    - To determine the etiology and severity of chronic liver disease (staging fibrosis, grading inflammation).
    - To diagnose infiltrative diseases (granulomatous diseases, amyloidosis, haemochromatosis).
    - To differentiate between benign and malignant liver lesions.
    - To assess drug-induced liver injury.
    - To guide treatment decisions and monitor disease progression.

- Types of Liver Biopsy:
  - Percutaneous Liver Biopsy: Most common approach, needle inserted through the skin into the liver under imaging guidance (ultrasound or CT).
  - Trans jugular Liver Biopsy: Needle advanced through the jugular vein into the hepatic vein to obtain liver tissue, preferred in patients with coagulopathy or ascites.
  - Laparoscopic Liver Biopsy: Performed during laparoscopy, allows for direct visualization and targeted biopsy, useful for focal lesions or when percutaneous approach is contraindicated.

Comparative Summary Framework for Differential Diagnosis

By organizing our thinking around these categories, we can construct a framework that helps in systematically narrowing down the differential diagnosis. Here's a conceptual representation of how such a framework can be visualized and utilized:

Category of Hepatomegaly	Common Causes	Key Presentations	Diagnostic Clues	Key Investigations
Congestive Hepatomegaly	Right-sided Heart Failure, Constrictive Pericarditis, Tricuspid Regurgitation, Budd-Chiari Syndrome, Veno-occlusive Disease	Peripheral edema, Jugular Venous Distension (JVD), Ascites, Hepatomegaly often tender, May have cardiac symptoms (dyspnea, fatigue)	History of heart disease, Elevated JVP, Lower extremity edema, Hepatojugular reflux	Echocardiogram, Liver Function Tests (LFTs) - often mildly elevated, Abdominal Ultrasound with Doppler (assess hepatic veins), BNP/NT-proBNP levels
Infiltrative Hepatomegaly	Malignancy (Metastatic Cancer, Lymphoma, Leukaemia), Amyloidosis, Sarcoidosis, Myeloproliferative Neoplasms	Variable - may be asymptomatic initially, Weight loss, Fatigue, Night sweats, Fever, Hepatomegaly often firm/nodular, May have extrahepatic manifestations (e.g., skin lesions in sarcoidosis)	History of malignancy, Unexplained weight loss, Systemic symptoms, Abnormal blood counts	Full Blood Count, LFTs - may be variably affected, Imaging (CT/ MRI abdomen) to assess for masses, Liver Biopsy (essential for definitive diagnosis in most cases)

Inflammatory Hepatomegaly	Viral Hepatitis (A, B, C, E, EBV, CMV), Autoimmune Hepatitis, Alcoholic Hepatitis, Drug-Induced Liver Injury (DILI), Primary Biliary Cholangitis (PBC), Primary Sclerosing Cholangitis (PSC)	Jaundice, Fatigue, Nausea/ Vomiting, Abdominal pain (RUQ), Pruritus (itching), Hepatomegaly often tender, May have features of chronic liver disease in prolonged cases	Risk factors for viral hepatitis, History of alcohol abuse, Medication history, Autoimmune features (e.g., joint pain, rash)	Viral Hepatitis Serology, Autoimmune Markers (ANA, ASMA, anti-LKM1 etc.), LFTs - often significantly elevated, Liver Ultrasound (rule out biliary obstruction), Consider Liver Biopsy
Metabolic/ Storage Hepatomegaly	Non-Alcoholic Fatty Liver Disease (NAFLD)/ Non-Alcoholic Steatohepatitis (NASH), Haemochromatosis, Wilson's Disease, Glycogen Storage Diseases, Lysosomal Storage Diseases	Often asymptomatic initially (NAFLD/NASH), Fatigue, Abdominal discomfort, Features of metabolic syndrome (obesity, diabetes, hyperlipidemia), Specific findings depending on the storage disease (e.g., Kayser-Fleischer rings in Wilson's, skin pigmentation in haemochromatosis)	Obesity, Diabetes, Hyperlipidaemia, Family history of metabolic/ storage disorders, Elevated ferritin (Haemochromatosis), Neurological symptoms (Wilson's)	LFTs - often mildly elevated in NAFLD/ NASH, Liver Ultrasound (fatty liver), Iron Studies (Haemochromatosis), Copper Studies (Wilson's), Genetic testing (for specific storage diseases), Consider Liver Biopsy (NAFLD/NASH staging)

Neoplastic Hepatomegaly	Hepatocellular Carcinoma (HCC), Cholangiocarcinoma, Hepatic Adenoma, Hemangioma (often benign, but can cause hepatomegaly), Liver Metastases	May be asymptomatic initially, Abdominal pain, Weight loss, Jaundice (in advanced cases), Palpable liver mass, Ascites, Features of chronic liver disease (in HCC arising in cirrhosis)	Risk factors for HCC (chronic viral hepatitis, cirrhosis), History of malignancy, Palpable mass, Elevated AFP (HCC), New onset or worsening ascites	LFTs - variably affected, AFP levels, Liver Ultrasound, Multiphasic CT or MRI of the Liver (essential for characterization), Liver Biopsy (often needed for definitive diagnosis and grading)
Biliary/ Obstructive Hepatomegaly	Choledocholithiasis, Biliary Strictures (benign or malignant), Cholangiocarcinoma (intrahepatic and extrahepatic), Primary Sclerosing Cholangitis (PSC)	Jaundice, Pruritus, Dark urine, Pale stools, Abdominal pain (RUQ), Fever/Chills (if cholangitis), Hepatomegaly often smooth and firm	History of gallstones, Elevated bilirubin and alkaline phosphatase, Symptoms of cholestasis (jaundice, pruritus), Imaging showing biliary dilatation	LFTs - Elevated bilirubin and alkaline phosphatase predominantly, Liver Ultrasound (assess biliary tree), MRCP/ ERCP (to visualize biliary ducts and identify obstruction), CT abdomen (to evaluate for mass lesions)

Differential Diagnosis of Jaundice

Introduction

Jaundice, clinically manifest as a yellowish discoloration of the skin, sclera, and mucous membranes, is a cardinal sign of underlying hepatobiliary disease and systemic disorders impacting bilirubin metabolism. While often visually striking and alarming to patients, jaundice itself is merely a symptom, a visible manifestation of elevated serum bilirubin levels. Understanding the complex pathways of bilirubin production, conjugation, and excretion is paramount to unravelling the diverse etiologies of jaundice. This chapter will delve into the differential diagnosis of jaundice, exploring the key presentations, diagnostic approaches, and providing a comparative summary to aid clinicians in navigating this common yet intricate clinical challenge.

Understanding Bilirubin Metabolism: A Foundation for Differential Diagnosis

Before embarking on the differential diagnosis, a brief review of bilirubin metabolism is crucial. Bilirubin, a tetrapyrrole pigment, is primarily derived from the breakdown of heme, predominantly from senescent red blood cells in the reticuloendothelial system (spleen, liver, bone marrow). This process yields unconjugated bilirubin, which is water-insoluble and transported in the plasma bound to albumin. The liver plays the central role in bilirubin metabolism. Hepatocytes uptake unconjugated bilirubin, conjugate it with glucuronic acid via uridine diphosphate glucuronosyltransferase 1A1 (UGT1A1), rendering it water-soluble (conjugated bilirubin). Conjugated bilirubin is then actively excreted into the bile canaliculi, contributing to bile. Bile flows through the biliary tree into the gallbladder and eventually the duodenum. In the gut, bacterial enzymes deconjugate bilirubin and convert it into urobilinogen. Urobilinogen are partly reabsorbed into the enterohepatic circulation, with a small fraction excreted in the urine and the remainder in the feces, providing the characteristic color to both.

Disruptions at any point in this intricate pathway can lead to hyperbilirubinemia and subsequent jaundice. Broadly, jaundice can be categorized into three main types based on the primary defect:

- Pre-hepatic (Haemolytic) Jaundice: Caused by excessive bilirubin production due to accelerated haemolysis. The liver's capacity to conjugate bilirubin is overwhelmed.
- Hepatic (Hepatocellular) Jaundice: Arises from intrinsic liver disease impairing bilirubin uptake, conjugation, and excretion. Hepatocellular dysfunction is the primary culprit.
- Post-hepatic (Obstructive) Jaundice: Results from obstruction of bile flow within the biliary tree, preventing conjugated bilirubin excretion into the intestine.

Key Presentations of Jaundice: Clues from the Clinical Picture

The clinical presentation of jaundice can vary dramatically depending on the underlying etiology. A careful history and physical examination, coupled with astute observation of associated symptoms, are crucial for narrowing the differential diagnosis.

1. Pre-hepatic Jaundice (Haemolytic):

- Presentation:
    - Subtle Jaundice: Often mild or moderate, may be easily missed initially, particularly in individuals with darker skin tones.
    - Absence of Dark Urine (or mildly tea-colored): Due to the excess bilirubin being primarily unconjugated and water-insoluble, less bilirubin is excreted in the urine.
    - Normal or Pale Stools: Bile flow into the intestine is not significantly obstructed, hence stool color is usually normal or may be slightly pale due to rapid transit.

- Splenomegaly: Often present due to increased red blood cell destruction in the spleen.
- Signs of Anemia: Pallor, fatigue, tachycardia, shortness of breath may accompany jaundice, reflecting the underlying haemolytic Anemia.
- Absence of Pruritus: Itching is typically not a prominent feature in pre-hepatic jaundice.
- Dark Urine Upon Standing (due to urobilinogen): Although initially not dark, urine might darken upon standing due to the oxidation of increased urinary urobilinogen.

- Key Historical Clues:
  - Family History of Haemolytic Anemia: Genetic conditions like sickle cell anemia, thalassemia, glucose-6-phosphate dehydrogenase (G6PD) deficiency, and hereditary spherocytosis should be considered.
  - Medications: Certain drugs can trigger haemolysis, such as sulfonamides, nitrofurantoin, and quinine in G6PD deficient individuals.
  - Recent Transfusion Reaction: Haemolytic transfusion reactions can lead to pre-hepatic jaundice.
  - Underlying Systemic Illnesses: Autoimmune haemolytic anemia can be associated with autoimmune disorders like systemic lupus erythematosus (SLE) or lymphoma.

2. Hepatic Jaundice (Hepatocellular):

- Presentation:
  - Moderate to Marked Jaundice: Often more pronounced than pre-hepatic jaundice, with readily apparent yellowing of sclera and skin.
  - Dark Urine (Tea-colored or Cola-colored): Conjugated bilirubin, which is water-soluble, is excreted in excess in the urine due to impaired hepatic excretion.

- Normal or Pale Stools: Stool color can be variable, ranging from normal to pale, depending on the severity of intrahepatic cholestasis and bile excretion impairment.
- Hepatomegaly: Liver enlargement may be present and tender, especially in acute hepatitis.
- Signs of Liver Dysfunction:
    - Fatigue and Malaise: Common non-specific symptoms.
    - Nausea and Vomiting: Especially in acute hepatitis.
    - Abdominal Pain: Right upper quadrant discomfort or diffuse abdominal pain may occur.
    - Ascites: Fluid accumulation in the abdomen in chronic liver disease and cirrhosis.
    - Edema: Peripheral edema due to hypoalbuminemia in chronic liver disease.
    - Coagulopathy: Increased risk of bleeding and bruising due to impaired synthesis of clotting factors.
    - Hepatic Encephalopathy: Altered mental status, confusion, asterixis in advanced liver failure.
- Pruritus: Itching can be present but is generally less prominent compared to post-hepatic jaundice.

- Key Historical Clues:
    - History of Viral Hepatitis Exposure: Hepatitis A, B, C, D, E infections. Risk factors include injection drug use, unprotected sexual activity, travel to endemic areas, and healthcare work.
    - Alcohol History: Chronic alcohol abuse can lead to alcoholic hepatitis and cirrhosis.
    - Medication History: Drug-induced liver injury (DILI) is a significant cause of hepatic jaundice. Many medications can cause hepatotoxicity.

- Non-Alcoholic Fatty Liver Disease (NAFLD) Risk Factors: Obesity, diabetes, hyperlipidemia, metabolic syndrome.
- Autoimmune Disease History: Autoimmune hepatitis, primary biliary cholangitis (PBC), primary sclerosing cholangitis (PSC).
- Genetic Liver Disease History: Wilson disease, haemochromatosis, alpha-1 antitrypsin deficiency.
- Travel History: Exposure to hepatitis viruses in endemic regions.
- Blood Transfusion History (Prior to screening): Risk factor for hepatitis B and C.

3. Post-hepatic Jaundice (Obstructive):

- Presentation:
  - Marked and Progressive Jaundice: Often deep yellow or even greenish-yellow, progressively worsening.
  - Dark Urine (Cola-colored): Conjugated bilirubin is regurgitated into the bloodstream and excreted in large amounts in the urine.
  - Pale or Clay-colored Stools (Acholic stools): Bile flow into the intestine is significantly reduced or completely obstructed, resulting in pale stools.
  - Pruritus (Intense Itching): A hallmark symptom, often severe and debilitating, attributed to bile salt accumulation in the skin.
  - Right Upper Quadrant Pain (RUQ pain): Biliary colic due to gallstones, or constant pain in pancreatic cancer or cholangitis.
  - Fever and Chills (if cholangitis present): Infections ascending the biliary tree can lead to acute cholangitis.
  - Weight Loss and Anorexia (in malignant obstruction): Particularly in pancreatic cancer or cholangiocarcinoma.

- Palpable Gallbladder (Courvoisier's Sign): In painless jaundice due to pancreatic cancer obstructing the distal common bile duct.
- Hepatomegaly (Variable): May be present, especially if prolonged obstruction leads to secondary biliary cirrhosis.

- Key Historical Clues:
    - Abdominal Pain History: Biliary colic, history of gallstones.
    - Risk Factors for Gallstones: Female gender, obesity, rapid weight loss, pregnancy, family history.
    - Risk Factors for Pancreatic Cancer: Age over 55, smoking, diabetes, chronic pancreatitis, family history.
    - History of Inflammatory Bowel Disease (IBD): Increased risk of primary sclerosing cholangitis (PSC).
    - Prior Biliary Surgery or Instrumentation: Risk of biliary strictures.

Diagnostic Approaches: A Step-by-Step Algorithm

The diagnostic approach to jaundice should be systematic and stepwise, guided by the clinical presentation and initial laboratory investigations.

Step 1: History and Physical Examination:

- Detailed History: As outlined in the "Key Presentations" section, focus on:
    - Onset, duration, and progression of jaundice.
    - Associated symptoms: Pruritus, abdominal pain, dark urine, pale stools, fever, fatigue, weight loss.
    - Past medical history: Liver disease, haemolytic anemia, gallstones, IBD, malignancy, diabetes, obesity, autoimmune disorders.
    - Medications, alcohol, and drug history (including herbal supplements).
    - Family history of jaundice or liver disease.
    - Travel history and exposure to risk factors for viral hepatitis.

- Thorough Physical Examination:
  - Assess the degree and distribution of jaundice (sclera, skin, mucous membranes).
  - Evaluate for hepatomegaly, splenomegaly, abdominal tenderness, ascites, peripheral edema.
  - Look for signs of chronic liver disease (spider angiomata, palmar erythema, gynecomastia, testicular atrophy).
  - Assess for lymphadenopathy and signs of systemic illness.
  - Palpate for gallbladder (Courvoisier's sign).

Step 2: Initial Laboratory Investigations:

- Liver Function Tests (LFTs):
  - Total Bilirubin and Direct Bilirubin (Conjugated): Essential for confirming hyperbilirubinemia and differentiating conjugated from unconjugated hyperbilirubinemia.
  - Aspartate Aminotransferase (AST) and Alanine Aminotransferase (ALT): Markers of hepatocellular injury. Elevated in hepatic jaundice, often dramatically increased in acute hepatitis.
  - Alkaline Phosphatase (ALP) and Gamma-Glutamyl Transferase (GGT): Markers of cholestasis (bile flow obstruction). Predominantly elevated in post-hepatic jaundice and intrahepatic cholestasis. GGT helps confirm liver origin of elevated ALP.
  - Albumin: Reduced in chronic liver disease reflecting impaired synthetic function.
  - Prothrombin Time (PT) / INR: Prolonged in severe liver disease due to impaired synthesis of clotting factors.
- Complete Blood Count (CBC):
  - Haemoglobin and Hematocrit: Assess for anemia, especially in pre-hepatic jaundice.

- Reticulocyte Count: Elevated in haemolytic anemia.
- Peripheral Blood Smear: Evaluate for morphological abnormalities of red blood cells suggesting haemolytic disorders (e.g., spherocytes in hereditary spherocytosis, sickle cells in sickle cell anemia).

- Urinalysis:
    - Urine Bilirubin: Positive in conjugated hyperbilirubinemia (hepatic and post-hepatic jaundice), negative or weakly positive in unconjugated hyperbilirubinemia (pre-hepatic jaundice).
    - Urine Urobilinogen: Increased in pre-hepatic jaundice and early hepatic jaundice, decreased or absent in complete biliary obstruction (post-hepatic jaundice).

Step 3: Interpreting LFT Patterns and Guiding Further Investigations:

The pattern of LFT abnormalities helps differentiate the three major categories of jaundice:

- Predominantly Unconjugated Hyperbilirubinemia (Unconjugated Bilirubin > 80% of Total Bilirubin): Suggests pre-hepatic jaundice.
    - Normal AST, ALT, ALP, GGT: Typically seen in Gilbert's syndrome (mild, isolated unconjugated hyperbilirubinemia).
    - Elevated Reticulocyte Count, Anemia: Suggests haemolytic anemia. Further investigations include:
        - Direct Antiglobulin Test (DAT) – Coombs test: To evaluate for autoimmune haemolytic anemia.
        - Haemoglobin Electrophoresis: To rule out haemoglobinopathies (thalassemia, sickle cell anemia).
        - G6PD Assay: To assess for G6PD deficiency.
        - Peripheral Blood Smear Review: For red cell morphology.

- Mixed Hyperbilirubinemia (Both Conjugated and Unconjugated Bilirubin Elevated): Suggests hepatic jaundice.
    - Elevated AST, ALT (often much higher than ALP): Hepatocellular injury predominant. Consider viral hepatitis, DILI, alcoholic hepatitis, autoimmune hepatitis, NAFLD/NASH.
        - Viral Hepatitis Serology: Hepatitis A, B, C, D, E virus panels.
        - Autoimmune Hepatitis Markers: Anti-nuclear antibody (ANA), anti-smooth muscle antibody (ASMA), anti-liver-kidney microsomal type 1 antibody (anti-LKM1), immunoglobulin levels.
        - Alcohol History and Biomarkers: Evaluate for alcoholic liver disease.
        - Medication History Review and DILI workup.
        - Ferritin and Transferrin Saturation: Screen for haemochromatosis.
        - Ceruloplasmin: Screen for Wilson disease (especially in young patients).
- Elevated ALP, GGT (often higher than AST, ALT): Cholestatic pattern within hepatic jaundice. Consider intrahepatic cholestasis of pregnancy, primary biliary cholangitis (PBC), primary sclerosing cholangitis (PSC), drug-induced cholestasis, infiltrative liver diseases (e.g., sarcoidosis, amyloidosis).
        - Antimitochondrial Antibody (AMA): For PBC.
        - Magnetic Resonance Cholangiopancreatography (MRCP) or Endoscopic Retrograde Cholangiopancreatography (ERCP): To evaluate for PSC and exclude extrahepatic obstruction.
        - Liver Biopsy: May be necessary to confirm diagnosis and assess disease severity in many hepatic conditions (e.g., autoimmune hepatitis, PBC, PSC, NAFLD/NASH, DILI).

- Predominantly Conjugated Hyperbilirubinemia (Conjugated Bilirubin > 50% of Total Bilirubin): Suggests post-hepatic jaundice.
    - Markedly Elevated ALP, GGT (often disproportionately higher than AST, ALT): Obstructive cholestasis.
        - Abdominal Ultrasound: Initial imaging modality to detect gallstones, biliary dilatation.
        - Computed Tomography (CT) Scan of Abdomen and Pelvis: To further evaluate for pancreatic masses, biliary tumors, lymphadenopathy, assess biliary tree anatomy.
        - Magnetic Resonance Cholangiopancreatography (MRCP): Excellent for visualizing biliary ducts and identifying strictures, stones, or tumors. Often preferred over ERCP as non-invasive.
        - Endoscopic Ultrasound (EUS): Useful for evaluating pancreatic lesions, distal bile duct, and ampulla of Vater.
        - Endoscopic Retrograde Cholangiopancreatography (ERCP): Both diagnostic and therapeutic; can visualize biliary tree, obtain biopsies, and perform biliary drainage (stenting). Reserved for cases where MRCP is inconclusive or therapeutic intervention is needed.

Step 4: Advanced Investigations and Liver Biopsy:

Depending on the clinical picture and initial investigations, further specialized tests may be required:

- Liver Biopsy: Gold standard for diagnosing and staging many hepatic diseases (autoimmune hepatitis, NAFLD/NASH, PBC, PSC, DILI, infiltrative diseases). Can help differentiate between hepatocellular and cholestatic patterns of injury and assess fibrosis.
- ERCP or Percutaneous Transhepatic Cholangiography (PTC): For further evaluation and therapeutic intervention in obstructive jaundice when non-invasive imaging is inadequate.

- Genetic Testing: For suspected genetic liver diseases (Gilbert's syndrome, Crigler-Najjar syndrome, Dubin-Johnson syndrome, Rotor syndrome, Wilson disease, haemochromatosis, alpha-1 antitrypsin deficiency).

Comparative summary table

Feature	**Pre-Hepatic Jaundice (Haemolytic)**	**Hepatic Jaundice (Hepatocellular)**	**Post-Hepatic Jaundice (Obstructive)**	**Neonatal Jaundice (Physiological/ Pathological)**
Primary Cause	Excessive Red Blood Cell Breakdown (Haemolysis)	Liver Cell Damage or Dysfunction	Obstruction of Bile Flow	Immature Liver Function & Increased RBC Breakdown in Newborns
Location of Problem	Before the Liver	Within the Liver	After the Liver (Bile Ducts)	Liver and Bilirubin Processing in Newborns
Bilirubin Type Predominantly Elevated	Unconjugated (Indirect) Bilirubin	Both Conjugated (Direct) and Unconjugated Bilirubin	Conjugated (Direct) Bilirubin	Primarily Unconjugated Bilirubin (Initially)
Urine Color	Normal or Darker Amber	Dark (Tea-colored)	Dark (Tea-colored)	Normal to Darker Amber (Depending on Severity)
Stool Color	Normal Color	Normal or Pale Color	Pale or Clay-colored	Normal to Pale Color (Depending on Cause)
Liver Enzymes (AST/ALT)	Usually Normal or Mildly Elevated	Often Elevated (Significantly)	Mildly Elevated or Normal	Usually Normal to Mildly Elevated

Common Causes	Haemolytic Anemias (e.g., Sickle Cell, G6PD Deficiency), Malaria, Blood Transfusion Reactions	Viral Hepatitis, Alcoholic Liver Disease, Cirrhosis, Autoimmune Hepatitis, Drug-Induced Liver Injury, Genetic Disorders (e.g., Gilbert's Syndrome)	Gallstones in Bile Ducts, Tumors in Bile Ducts or Pancreas, Biliary Strictures, Primary Sclerosing Cholangitis	Physiological Jaundice (Normal Newborn), Breast Milk Jaundice, Blood Group Incompatibility (Rh or ABO), Prematurity, Infections, Genetic Disorders
Key Clinical Features	Splenomegaly (enlarged spleen), Anemia signs, No significant bilirubinuria	Fatigue, Nausea, Abdominal pain, Pale stools (sometimes), Pruritus (itching), Bilirubinuria	Severe Pruritus, Pale stools ("acholic stools"), Dark urine, Abdominal pain, Jaundice often progresses	Jaundice appearing within first few days of life, Poor feeding, Lethargy (in severe cases), Kernicterus risk (in severe unconjugated hyperbilirubinemia)
Treatment Focus	Treat Underlying Cause (e.g., Blood transfusion, manage haemolytic condition)	Treat Underlying Liver Disease (e.g., Antivirals, Alcohol abstinence, Immunosuppressants), Liver support, Liver Transplant (in severe cases)	Relieve Bile Duct Obstruction (Surgical removal of gallstones, Stenting of bile ducts, Tumor resection), Treat underlying cause	Phototherapy (most common), Exchange Transfusion (severe unconjugated hyperbilirubinemia), Treat underlying cause (e.g., infection, blood group incompatibility)

Differential Diagnosis of Portal Hypertension

Introduction

Portal hypertension, defined as an elevated pressure gradient between the portal vein and the hepatic vein (typically >5 mmHg), is a cardinal manifestation of chronic liver disease and other conditions affecting the hepatic circulation. While cirrhosis is undeniably the most common cause in developed nations, portal hypertension is not synonymous with cirrhosis. A spectrum of underlying etiologies, ranging from pre-hepatic to intrahepatic and post-hepatic vascular obstructions, can lead to this critical pathophysiological state. Furthermore, the clinical consequences of portal hypertension – variceal haemorrhage, ascites, hepatic encephalopathy, and hepatorenal syndrome – represent significant morbidity and mortality drivers in patients with liver disease.

Accurate differential diagnosis of portal hypertension is paramount for effective management. Identifying the underlying cause is crucial not only for tailoring specific treatments to address the root pathology but also for stratifying risk, predicting prognosis, and guiding decisions regarding transplantation. This chapter delves into the intricate landscape of differential diagnosis for portal hypertension, exploring the key clinical presentations, diagnostic approaches, and comparative features that allow clinicians to navigate this complex clinical challenge. We will examine the diverse spectrum of etiologies, from common culprits to rarer conditions, equipping the reader with a comprehensive framework for approaching patients with suspected or confirmed portal hypertension.

Key Presentations of Portal Hypertension

Portal hypertension itself is often clinically silent in its early stages. Many patients may remain asymptomatic until complications arise. However, understanding the potential presenting features is essential for early suspicion and timely diagnosis. The clinical manifestations of portal hypertension are primarily attributable to two intertwined pathophysiological mechanisms: the increased pressure gradient within the portal system and the development of portosystemic shunts.

Common Presentations:

- Variceal Bleeding (Hematemesis and/or Melena): This is often the most dramatic and life-threatening presentation. Increased portal pressure leads to the development of portosystemic collaterals, most notably esophageal and gastric varices. Rupture of these fragile varices results in upper gastrointestinal bleeding, manifesting as hematemesis (vomiting blood, often described as "coffee-ground" emesis) and melena (black, tarry stools). Variceal bleeding is a medical emergency requiring prompt resuscitation and intervention.
- Ascites: The accumulation of fluid in the peritoneal cavity is a common and debilitating complication of portal hypertension. Ascites develops due to a complex interplay of factors including splanchnic vasodilation, renal sodium and water retention, decreased oncotic pressure (hypoalbuminemia), and increased hepatic lymph production. Clinically, ascites presents as progressive abdominal distension, weight gain, and abdominal discomfort. In severe cases, it can cause respiratory distress and contribute to spontaneous bacterial peritonitis (SBP).
- Splenomegaly: Increased portal pressure leads to congestion of the spleen, resulting in splenomegaly (enlarged spleen). While often asymptomatic, splenomegaly can be detected on physical examination as a palpable spleen below the left costal margin. It can contribute to hypersplenism, leading to thrombocytopenia, leukopenia, and anemia.
- Hepatic Encephalopathy: This neuropsychiatric syndrome is a consequence of liver dysfunction and portosystemic shunting. Failure of the liver to detoxify neurotoxins, particularly ammonia, allows these substances to bypass the liver and reach the brain. Hepatic encephalopathy manifests as a spectrum of neurological

and cognitive abnormalities, ranging from subtle changes in personality, sleep disturbances, and impaired concentration to overt confusion, asterixis (flapping tremor), and coma. Episodes can be precipitated by factors like gastrointestinal bleeding, infection, constipation, and electrolyte imbalances.

Less Frequent or Subtle Presentations:

- Caput Medusae: Distended superficial abdominal veins radiating outwards from the umbilicus, creating a "Medusa's head" appearance. This is a visible sign of portosystemic collateralization, although less common in contemporary practice due to earlier diagnosis.
- Haemorrhoids: While haemorrhoids are common in the general population, portal hypertension can exacerbate or contribute to haemorrhoidal dilatation due to increased pressure in the inferior rectal veins, which are part of the portosystemic circulation.
- Thrombocytopenia and Leukopenia: Hypersplenism secondary to splenomegaly can lead to decreased platelet and white blood cell counts, which may be detected incidentally on routine blood tests.
- Unexplained Abdominal Pain or Discomfort: Some patients may experience vague abdominal discomfort or pain due to liver congestion or splenomegaly, although this is a non-specific symptom.
- Jaundice (Icterus): While jaundice is primarily a sign of hepatic dysfunction, it can be associated with portal hypertension, especially in the context of underlying liver disease.

It is crucial to remember that the presentation of portal hypertension can be highly variable and depends on the underlying etiology, the severity of the disease, and the presence of complications. A high index of suspicion is essential, particularly in patients with known risk factors for liver disease or presenting with any of the aforementioned symptoms.

Diagnostic Approaches to Portal Hypertension

The diagnostic evaluation of portal hypertension aims to confirm its presence, identify the underlying cause, assess the severity, and detect any associated complications. A stepwise approach, combining clinical assessment, laboratory investigations, imaging modalities, and in some cases, invasive procedures, is typically employed.

1. Clinical Assessment:

- History: A thorough medical history is vital, focusing on:
    - Risk factors for liver disease: Alcohol consumption, viral hepatitis (B and C), non-alcoholic fatty liver disease (NAFLD) risk factors (obesity, diabetes, hyperlipidemia), autoimmune diseases, medications (e.g., methotrexate, amiodarone), family history of liver disease.
    - Symptoms of liver disease and portal hypertension: History of jaundice, ascites, variceal bleeding, encephalopathy, fatigue, abdominal pain, weight changes.
    - History of thrombophilia, myeloproliferative disorders, or other conditions predisposing to vascular thromboses (for pre-hepatic and post-hepatic causes).
    - History of cardiac disease (for post-hepatic causes like constrictive pericarditis or right heart failure).
    - Medication history, including potential hepatotoxic drugs and anticoagulants.

- Physical Examination: A comprehensive physical exam should include:
    - General appearance: Assess for signs of chronic liver disease such as jaundice, muscle wasting, spider angiomata, palmar erythema, gynecomastia, and parotid gland enlargement.
    - Abdominal examination: Palpate for hepatomegaly, splenomegaly, ascites (shifting dullness, fluid wave), and abdominal tenderness. Inspect for caput medusae.

  - Neurological examination: Assess for signs of hepatic encephalopathy (mental status changes, asterixis, hyperreflexia).
  - Cardiovascular examination: Evaluate for signs of right heart failure (jugular venous distension, peripheral edema) or constrictive pericarditis (Kussmaul's sign, pericardial knock).

2. Laboratory Investigations:

- Liver Function Tests (LFTs): Alanine aminotransferase (ALT), aspartate aminotransferase (AST), alkaline phosphatase (ALP), bilirubin (total and direct), albumin, prothrombin time/INR. These tests provide information about liver inflammation, synthetic function, and cholestasis. While abnormal in most causes of portal hypertension, the pattern and degree of abnormality can vary depending on the underlying etiology.
- Complete Blood Count (CBC): To assess for thrombocytopenia, leukopenia, and anemia, which can be indicative of hypersplenism and/or bone marrow suppression in advanced liver disease.
- Renal Function Tests: Serum creatinine, blood urea nitrogen (BUN), electrolytes (sodium, potassium). Important for assessing for hepatorenal syndrome and monitoring renal function, especially in patients with ascites and diuretics.
- Viral Hepatitis Serology: Testing for hepatitis B surface antigen (HBsAg), hepatitis B core antibody (anti-HBc), hepatitis C antibody (anti-HCV) and HCV RNA is crucial to identify viral hepatitis as a cause of liver disease and portal hypertension.
- Autoimmune Markers: Antinuclear antibodies (ANA), anti-smooth muscle antibodies (ASMA), anti-liver-kidney microsomal antibodies (anti-LKM1), anti-mitochondrial antibodies (AMA), immunoglobulin levels (IgG, IgA, IgM) to evaluate for autoimmune liver diseases as a potential cause.
- Iron Studies: Serum ferritin, transferrin saturation, total iron-binding capacity (TIBC) to assess for haemochromatosis.

- Alpha-1 Antitrypsin Level: To screen for alpha-1 antitrypsin deficiency.
- Ceruloplasmin and 24-hour Urinary Copper: To evaluate for Wilson's disease.
- Fasting Blood Glucose and Lipid Panel: To assess for metabolic syndrome and NAFLD risk factors.
- Coagulation Studies: Prothrombin time (PT), activated partial thromboplastin time (aPTT), fibrinogen, D-dimer. Used to assess liver synthetic function and identify hypercoagulable states (especially relevant in pre-hepatic and post-hepatic causes).
- Ascitic Fluid Analysis (if ascites is present): Cell count and differential, albumin, total protein, glucose, lactate dehydrogenase (LDH), Gram stain and culture, amylase, and cytology. Helps to diagnose SBP, exclude other causes of ascites, and assess the etiology of ascites.

3. Imaging Modalities:

- Abdominal Ultrasound (US) with Doppler: This is often the *first-line imaging modality* due to its non-invasiveness, availability, and cost-effectiveness.

    - Liver parenchyma: Assesses for echotexture changes suggestive of cirrhosis, fatty liver, or other liver diseases.
    - Portal vein: Evaluates portal vein diameter, patency (Doppler flow), direction of flow (hepatopetal vs. hepatofugal), and presence of thrombus.
    - Hepatic veins: Evaluates hepatic vein patency and flow patterns (important in Budd-Chiari syndrome).
    - Spleen: Measures splenic size to assess for splenomegaly.
    - Ascites: Detects and quantifies ascites.
    - Portosystemic collaterals: May visualize large collaterals, although sensitivity is limited.

- Computed Tomography (CT) Scan of the Abdomen with IV Contrast (CT Angiography): Provides more detailed anatomical information than ultrasound.
    - Liver parenchyma: better characterization of liver lesions, nodules, and masses.
    - Portal vein, hepatic veins, splenic vein, superior mesenteric vein: Excellent visualization of vascular anatomy and patency, detection of thrombosis, and assessment of collaterals.
    - Other abdominal organs: Evaluates for underlying malignancies, pancreatic disease, or other conditions that can contribute to portal hypertension.
- Magnetic Resonance Imaging (MRI) of the Abdomen with Gadolinium Contrast (MR Angiography/MR Venography): Offers superior soft tissue contrast and vascular imaging compared to CT, without ionizing radiation.
    - Liver parenchyma: Excellent characterization of liver lesions, including hepatocellular carcinoma (HCC).
    - Portal vein, hepatic veins, splenic vein, superior mesenteric vein: Provides detailed vascular anatomy and flow information, particularly valuable for diagnosing Budd-Chiari syndrome and portal vein thrombosis.
    - Diffusion-weighted imaging (DWI): Can be helpful in characterizing liver lesions.
- Liver Elastography (Fibro Scan or MR Elastography): Non-invasive assessment of liver stiffness, which correlates with liver fibrosis and portal hypertension severity in chronic liver diseases, particularly cirrhosis. Can help predict the presence of varices and complications.
- Hepatic Venous Pressure Gradient (HVPG) Measurement: This is an *invasive procedure* considered the "gold standard" for confirming the presence of portal hypertension and quantifying

its severity. A catheter is inserted percutaneously into the femoral or jugular vein, advanced into a hepatic vein, and pressure measurements are obtained. HVPG is calculated as the difference between wedged hepatic venous pressure (WHVP, reflecting sinusoidal pressure) and free hepatic venous pressure (FHVP, reflecting inferior vena cava pressure).

- Diagnostic: HVPG ≥ 5 mmHg confirms portal hypertension.
- Prognostic: HVPG ≥ 10 mmHg is associated with increased risk of variceal bleeding and other complications. HVPG ≥ 12 mmHg is generally considered clinically significant portal hypertension and a threshold for initiating prophylaxis and treatment.
- Research and clinical trials: HVPG is often used in clinical trials to assess the efficacy of interventions for portal hypertension.

- Endoscopy (Esophagogastroduodenoscopy - EGD): Essential for detecting esophageal and gastric varices, assessing their size and risk of bleeding (using endoscopic grading systems), and performing endoscopic variceal ligation (EVL) or sclerotherapy for primary or secondary prophylaxis of variceal bleeding.
- Liver Biopsy: While not routinely required for diagnosing portal hypertension *perse*, liver biopsy is crucial in many cases to determine the *underlying etiology* of liver disease causing portal hypertension, assess the degree of fibrosis, and exclude other liver pathologies. It is particularly important in differentiating between cirrhotic and non-cirrhotic causes of portal hypertension. However, liver biopsy is an invasive procedure with potential risks (bleeding, pain, infection) and may be contraindicated in patients with severe coagulopathy or ascites. Trans jugular liver biopsy can be considered in patients with coagulopathy or ascites, as it reduces the risk of bleeding complications compared to percutaneous biopsy.

4. Other Investigations (depending on clinical suspicion):

- Cardiac Echocardiography: To evaluate for right heart failure, constrictive pericarditis, or other cardiac causes of post-hepatic portal hypertension.
- Thrombophilia Screening: In cases of suspected portal vein thrombosis or Budd-Chiari syndrome, consider testing for hypercoagulable states (e.g., Factor V Leiden mutation, prothrombin gene mutation, antiphospholipid antibodies, protein C and S deficiency, antithrombin deficiency).
- Bone Marrow Biopsy: May be indicated in cases of suspected myeloproliferative disorders associated with Budd-Chiari syndrome.
- Genetic Testing: May be considered in selected cases to evaluate for genetic liver diseases (e.g., haemochromatosis, Wilson's disease, alpha-1 antitrypsin deficiency).

Comparative Summary:

Feature	**Pre-hepatic Portal Hypertension**	**Intra-hepatic Portal Hypertension**	**Post-hepatic Portal Hypertension**
Location of Obstruction	Portal vein/Splenic vein (Pre-liver)	Within the liver parenchyma (Liver)	Hepatic veins/IVC/Right Heart (Post-liver)
Typical Cause	Portal Vein Thrombosis (PVT)	Cirrhosis (various etiologies)	Budd-Chiari Syndrome (BCS), Right Heart Failure
Liver Function (Early)	Usually Preserved	Impaired	Initially Preserved, Progressively Impaired
Pathophysiology	Obstruction of inflow to liver	Increased resistance within liver	Obstruction of outflow from liver
Splenomegaly	Prominent, early feature	Variable, may be present	Hepatomegaly due to congestion, Splenomegaly may be present
Ascites	Less frequent, less severe initially	Frequent, often prominent and persistent	Frequent, often prominent
Jaundice	Less common initially	Common	Less common initially
Leg Edema/JVD	Less prominent	Less prominent	More prominent (especially in cardiac causes)
Key Diagnostic Clue	Imaging of portal vein (Doppler US, CT)	Liver biopsy, clinical signs of cirrhosis	Imaging of hepatic veins/IVC (Doppler US, CT/MRI)

Chapter Four

Musculoskeletal Diseases

Dr. Shriram Krishnamoorthy

Differential Diagnosis of Arthritis: A Comprehensive Review

Arthritis, a term that encompasses over 100 distinct inflammatory joint disorders, remains one of the leading causes of disability in the world. Accurate diagnosis is crucial for effective treatment and management, given that different types of arthritis can have similar symptoms but require widely varying treatment approaches. This article delves into the differential diagnosis of arthritis, highlighting key presentations, diagnostic approaches, a comparative summary, key takeaways, and concluding with a comprehensive bibliography inclusive of recent research.

Key Presentations of Arthritis

1. Joint Pain and Swelling

Joint pain and swelling are the hallmark symptoms of arthritis. The location (monoarthritis, oligoarthritis, or polyarthritis) and duration (acute or chronic) of symptoms can provide critical clues for diagnosis.

2. Stiffness

Morning stiffness lasting more than 30 minutes is characteristic of inflammatory arthritides, whereas stiffness that resolves within a few moments is more atypical.

3. Redness and Warmth

Erythema and increased temperature over the affected joints indicate active inflammation, which is often observed in conditions like gout and rheumatoid arthritis. *Associated with fever and other systemic symptoms septic arthritis can present with warmth.*

4. Decreased Range of Motion

Loss of range of motion is a critical presentation and can occur due to mechanical factors, inflammation, muscle spasms, or joint effusion.

5. Systemic Symptoms

Fever, fatigue, and weight loss are systemic signs that may accompany specific types of arthritis, such as systemic lupus erythematosus or inflammatory arthritis. *In Reactive arthritis / Reiter's syndrome arthritis is associated with uveitis and urethritis. In Psoriatic arthritis skin lesion are noticed.*

6. Extra-articular Manifestations

Certain arthritic conditions are associated with systemic manifestations, such as skin rashes in psoriasis, eye inflammation in reactive arthritis, or lung involvement in rheumatoid arthritis. *Tophi is noted in chronic gout (predominantly in 1st MTP)*

7. Crepitus

Crepitus is a crackling or grinding sensation felt or heard in a joint, and when associated with arthritis, it often indicates that the joint's articular cartilage has been eroded or roughened by conditions like osteoarthritis or rheumatoid arthritis. This sound occurs when two rough surfaces within the joint grind against each other during movement. While some joint noises are harmless, crepitus with pain, swelling, or stiffness can signal an underlying mechanical problem or active disease

Diagnostic Approaches

Clinical History

A thorough clinical history is paramount. The duration, onset, and character of symptoms, as well as family history and associated systemic symptoms, can guide clinicians toward an accurate diagnosis.

Physical Examination

Physical examination should focus on joint tenderness, swelling, range of motion, and extra-articular findings. The symmetric involvement of joints is particularly indicative of some inflammatory arthritides, such as rheumatoid arthritis.

Laboratory Tests

- Blood Tests: Various laboratory investigations can help distinguish between types of arthritis:
    - Rheumatoid Factor (RF): *Classical test for* rheumatoid arthritis *but low sensitivity.*
    - Anti-Cyclic Citrullinated Peptide (anti-CCP) Antibodies: More specific for rheumatoid arthritis.
    - Antinuclear Antibodies (ANA): Commonly associated with systemic lupus erythematosus and other connective tissue diseases.
    - Erythrocyte Sedimentation Rate (ESR) and C-Reactive Protein (CRP): Non-specific markers of inflammation often elevated in systemic inflammatory conditions.
    - *Uric acid is usually elevated in gouty arthritis*
- Synovial Fluid Analysis: Analyzing joint fluid can provide critical insights. Inflammatory arthritis often reveals increased white blood cell counts, whereas crystalline arthritis shows presence of crystals.
- Imaging Studies:
    - X-rays: Useful for assessing joint damage, erosions, and deformities.
    - *USG - Though highly user dependent can be handy in office to asses fluid volume and meniscal tears.*
    - MRI and Ultrasound: Advanced imaging techniques useful for detecting early joint inflammation and soft-tissue

involvement, especially in inflammatory arthritis. *Cartilogram is available these days as an extension to MRI to asses the thickness of articular cartilage. It can be especially useful to locate focal cartilage loss.*

- Genetic Testing: May help diagnose conditions with a genetic component, such as Ankylosing Spondylitis, often associated with HLA-B27 antigen.

Comparative Summary of Common Types of Arthritis

Type of Arthritis	**Key Presentations**	**Laboratory Findings**	**Imaging Findings**	**Treatment Approaches**
Rheumatoid Arthritis (RA)	Symmetrical polyarthritis, morning stiffness	Positive RF and anti-CCP antibodies	Joint erosions, deformities	DMARDs, NSAIDs, glucocorticoids. *Monoclonal antibodies*
Osteoarthritis (OA)	Joint pain with activity, crepitus	Normal RF, ESR and CRP typically low	Joint space narrowing, osteophytes	Analgesics, physical therapy, *intaarticular injection, surgical intervention like Knee replacement.*
Gout	Sudden onset, monoarthritis (especially big toe)	Elevated uric acid, presence of crystals	Normal or acute inflammation signs	NSAIDs, colchicine, urate-lowering therapy
Psoriatic Arthritis (PsA)	Nail changes, dactylitis, asymmetric joints	Positive ANA, possible RF	Erosive changes, pencil-in-cup deformity	DMARDs, TNF inhibitors
Ankylosing Spondylitis (AS)	Inflammatory back pain, morning stiffness	Positive HLA-B27	Sacroiliitis on X-ray, fusion over time	NSAIDs, physiotherapy, TNF inhibitors, *Monoclonal antibodies.*

Key Takeaways

- Comprehensive Evaluation: arthritis diagnosis requires a careful evaluation of clinical symptoms, physical examination, and laboratory assessments to differentiate between the various forms of the disease.
- Importance of Early Diagnosis: Understanding the nuances in presentations can precipitate timely intervention, significantly impacting long-term outcomes.
- Multi-disciplinary Approach: Collaboration with rheumatologists, physiotherapists, and other specialists is important for holistic management of patients with arthritis.
- Individualized Treatment Plans: Tailoring treatment plans based on the specific type of arthritis, severity, and patient preferences is crucial in optimal management.
- Ongoing Research: Continual advancements in the understanding of the pathogenesis and treatment options are helping improve outcomes for arthritis patients.

Summary

The differential diagnosis of arthritis is complex and requires a comprehensive understanding of various types, clinical presentations, and resourceful diagnostic methodologies. A timely and accurate diagnosis can significantly influence the prognosis and quality of life for individuals suffering from this often-debilitating condition. Ongoing research is vital in achieving better understanding and targeting effective interventions.

Bibliography

- Kryczka, J., et al. "Differential Diagnosis of Arthritis in Daily Practice." *Clinical Rheumatology*, vol. 42, no. 11, 2023, pp. 4731-4746.
- Richette, P., & Bardin, T. "Gout." *The Lancet*, vol. 392, no. 10156, 2018, pp. 1875–87.

- Aletaha, D., & Smolen, J. S. "The ACR/EULAR 2010 Rheumatoid Arthritis Classification Criteria: An American College of Rheumatology/European League Against Rheumatism Collaborative Initiative." *Arthritis & Rheumatism*, vol. 62, no. 9, 2010, pp. 2569-2581.
- Inman, R. D., & Alavi, A. "Ankylosing Spondylitis and Related Disorders." *The New England Journal of Medicine*, vol. 388, no. 25, 2023, pp. 2418-2430.
- Pellets, T., et al. "Management of Psoriatic Arthritis." *Rheumatology*, vol. 62, no. 4, 2023, pp. 839-845.
- Hunter, D. J., & Felson, D. T. "Osteoarthritis." *BMJ*, vol. 333, no. 7570, 2006, pp. 626-631.
- Negm, A., et al. "Update on the Prevention and Treatment of Gout." *Current Opinion in Rheumatology*, vol. 31, no. 2, 2023, pp. 147–155.
- Deodhar, A., et al. "The Role of IL-17 in Autoimmunity and Chronic Inflammation." *Nature Reviews Rheumatology*, vol. 14, no. 12, 2023, pp. 768–779.
- Bowe, A., & Harrington, J. "Update on the Diagnosis and Management of Rheumatoid Arthritis." *British Journal of General Practice*, vol. 73, no. 721, 2023, pp. 169-170.

Differential Diagnosis of Back Pain

Back pain is one of the most common health complaints among adults, affecting millions of people worldwide. With a complex array of potential causes, proper differential diagnosis is crucial to provide appropriate treatment and alleviate suffering. This article will explore key presentations of back pain, the diagnostic approaches employed, a comparative summary of various causes, key takeaways, and current perspectives based on recent research.

Key Presentations

When assessing back pain, it is essential to consider various presentations that may indicate different underlying conditions. Here are some key presentations:

1. Acute vs. Chronic Back Pain

- Acute Back Pain: Typically defined as pain lasting less than six weeks, acute back pain is often related to injury, strain, or inflammation. Patients may report sudden onset pain after lifting, sudden movements, or physical exertion.
- Chronic Back Pain: Defined as pain lasting longer than three months, chronic back pain often has multifactorial origins, including degenerative diseases, underlying medical conditions, or psychological factors.

2. Radicular Pain

Often associated with nerve root compression, radicular pain can present as sharp, shooting pain radiating down the legs. This is commonly due to herniated discs, spinal stenosis, or other causes of nerve irritation.

3. Mechanical Pain

Mechanical pain typically worsens with specific activities and improves when changing positions or resting. Conditions such as lumbar disc degeneration or spondylolisthesis are often involved.

4. Non-mechanical Pain

Non-mechanical causes of back pain often indicate serious underlying issues. This may include conditions such as infections, tumors, or systemic disorders like ankylosing spondylitis. These patients may report unremitting pain that is not responsive to rest or position changes.

5. Rest pain

Pain noticed after rest / early morning while waking up can usually be inflammatory arthritis like Rheumatoid and Ankylosing spondylitis.

6. Associated Symptoms

Back pain can be accompanied by other symptoms such as:

- Weakness or numbness in the legs
- Bowel or bladder dysfunction
- Fever or chills
- Unexplained weight loss

These accompanying symptoms can help direct the differential diagnosis process.

Diagnostic Approaches

An effective diagnostic approach to back pain begins with a comprehensive history and physical examination, followed by targeted investigations when indicated. Here are the common steps involved:

1. Patient History

The initial assessment involves gathering detailed information on the patient's pain characteristics:

- Onset: Acute or gradual.
- Duration: Current condition duration (acute vs chronic)
- Location: Localized or diffuse pain.
- Radiation: Pain that travels to other areas (e.g., legs).
- Factors: Activities that worsen or alleviate pain, presence of associated symptoms.

2. Physical Examination

A thorough physical examination includes:

- Inspection and Palpation: Assessing posture, spinal alignment, and tenderness.

- Range of Motion: Evaluating flexibility and limitations in movement.
- Neurological Examination: Checking reflexes, sensation, and muscle strength in the lower limbs to identify radiculopathy or other nerve-related conditions.

3. Imaging Studies

When physical examination findings and history suggest serious underlying causes or if symptoms persist, imaging studies may be warranted:

- X-rays: Useful for evaluating fractures, degenerative changes, and structural alignment.
- MRI: Provides detailed soft tissue imaging; essential for diagnosing disc herniation, spinal stenosis, or tumours.
- CT scans: Especially useful for assessing bony structures and complex spinal issues.

4. Laboratory Tests

Depending on the clinical suspicion, additional laboratory tests may be appropriate:

- Blood Tests: To rule out infection (like osteomyelitis) or autoimmune conditions (like ankylosing spondylitis).
- Urinalysis: To detect possible kidney stones if flank pain is present.

5. Referral to Specialists

For patients with complex or persistent cases, referral to specialists such as orthopaedic surgeons, neurologists, rheumatologists, or pain management specialists may be necessary. Multidisciplinary assessment can expand diagnostic possibilities and optimize treatment plans.

Comparative Summary of Causes of Back Pain

Here below is a comparative summary of common causes of back pain, categorized based on their clinical features, diagnostic considerations, and management approaches:

1. Musculoskeletal Causes

- Lumbar Strain/Sprain: Commonly due to heavy lifting or sudden movements; characterized by localized pain, tenderness, and spasm. Treatment focuses on rest, physiotherapy, and analgesics.
- Degenerative Disc Disease: Typically presents as chronic pain due to disc injury or degeneration; managed conservatively with physical therapy and medications, but surgery may be necessary in severe cases.

2. Neurological Causes

- Herniated Disc: Presentation includes radicular pain, sensory deficits, and motor weakness; MRI is critical for diagnosis. Treatment can include conservative management or surgical discectomy in severe cases.
- Spinal Stenosis: Patients often report leg pain that worsens with walking; imaging studies confirm diagnosis. Management can include physical therapy, epidural injections, or surgery.

3. Inflammatory Conditions

- Ankylosing Spondylitis (AS): Chronic back pain, morning stiffness, and improvement with exercise; diagnosed through clinical criteria and imaging (e.g., X-ray), often treated with NSAIDs.

4. Infective Causes

- Osteomyelitis or Discitis: Presents with pain, fever, and systemic symptoms; MRI and blood cultures are key for diagnosis. Treatment typically involves antibiotics and possibly surgical intervention.

5. Malignant Causes

- Metastatic Disease: Back pain with significant weight loss and other systemic symptoms; imaging and biopsy may be necessary for diagnosis. Approach usually requires multidisciplinary oncological care.

Key Takeaways

- Thorough Assessment is Key: A detailed patient history and physical examination are crucial for effective differential diagnosis of back pain.
- Identify Red Flags: Certain symptoms warrant urgent investigations, such as unexplained weight loss, bowel or bladder dysfunction, and severe neurological deficits.
- Multidisciplinary Approach: Complex back pain cases benefit significantly from evaluation by various specialists, ensuring comprehensive care.
- Individualized Management: Treatment options should be tailored to the underlying cause of back pain and the patient's unique circumstances, prioritizing non-invasive options where appropriate.

Comparative Summary

The following table provides a comparative summary of various conditions associated with back pain, their key presentations, common diagnostic approaches, and pertinent diagnostic findings.

Condition	Key Presentation	Common Diagnostic Approaches	Diagnostic Findings
Musculoskeletal Pain	Localized pain, stiffness	History and physical exam	Tenderness, muscle spasm
Radicular Pain	Shooting pain down the leg	MRI, nerve conduction studies	Positive straight leg raise test
Referred Pain	Dull ache with systemic symptoms	CBC, imaging based on organ	Normal back exam; organ-specific findings
Neuropathic Pain	Burning, tingling sensation	EMG, nerve conduction studies	Abnormal EMG results
Inflammatory Conditions	Morning stiffness	ESR, CRP, MRI	*FABER +ve,* Elevated ESR, inflammatory changes

Infectious Causes	Severe localized pain	CBC, MRI, blood cultures	Significantly elevated WBC count
Tumours	Persistent pain, night symptoms	MRI, CT scan	Mass on imaging, potential metastasis
Visceral Causes	Dull, nagging ache	Relevant organ imaging	Organ-specific pathology

Summary

The differential diagnosis of back pain is a multifaceted process that requires careful consideration of patient histories, clinical presentations, and appropriate diagnostic evaluations. By understanding the various causes of back pain and employing a systematic approach, healthcare providers can effectively identify underlying conditions and initiate the most appropriate treatment plans. Ongoing research continues to inform and enhance our understanding of back pain, underscoring the importance of evidence-based practice in effectively managing this prevalent condition.

Bibliography

- Atlas, S. J., & Deyo, R. A. (2011). *Evaluating and Managing Acute Low Back Pain in Adults.* JAMA.
- Chou, R., Yu, J., & Deyo, R. A. (2020). *Management of Low Back Pain.* BMJ.
- Riesgo, R. A., & Sapia, M. (2023). *Emerging Insights into Low Back Pain Management.* Current Pain and Headache Reports.
- Koes, B. W., van Tulder, M. W., & Thomas, S. (2018). *Diagnosis and Treatment of Low Back Pain.* BMJ.
- Steffens, D., et al. (2022). *Exercise and Back Pain: A Systematic Review of Randomized Controlled Trials.* Physical Therapy.

Differential Diagnosis of Connective Tissue Diseases (CTDs)

Connective tissue diseases (CTDs) are a broad group of disorders characterized by inflammation, degeneration, or malfunction of connective tissues, including collagen and elastin. These diseases involve a range of tissues such as skin, joints, muscles, blood vessels, and internal organs. Given their overlapping clinical manifestations, diagnosing a specific connective tissue disease remains a challenge. This article delves into the differential diagnosis of CTDs, focusing on key presentations, diagnostic approaches, a comparative summary, and practical takeaways.

Key Presentations

CTDs commonly present with systemic manifestations and multisystem involvement. While each disorder has hallmark features, shared symptoms make clinical distinction difficult, necessitating careful evaluation. Below are some hallmarks and overlapping symptoms seen in CTDs:

1. Systemic Lupus Erythematosus (SLE)

- Common Symptoms: Fever, fatigue, malar ("butterfly") rash, joint pain, oral ulcers, and photosensitivity. Severe cases may include kidney damage, neurological symptoms, and hematologic abnormalities.
- Hallmark Presentation: Multisystem involvement such as nephritis, pericarditis, or neurological disorders, often with antinuclear antibodies (ANA) as a key marker.

2. Rheumatoid Arthritis (RA)

- Common Symptoms: Symmetrical joint pain, stiffness (especially in the morning), and swelling, typically involving small joints.
- Hallmark Presentation: Synovitis with erosive arthritis visible in imaging studies, accompanied by positive rheumatoid factor (RF) or anti-citrullinated peptide antibodies (anti-CCP).

3. Systemic Sclerosis (Scleroderma)

- Common Symptoms: Skin tightening, Raynaud's phenomenon, digital ulcers, and dysphagia.

- Hallmark Presentation: Diffuse fibrosis of skin and internal organs (e.g., lungs, heart, gastrointestinal tract) along with anti-centromere antibodies in limited cutaneous forms or anti-Scl-70 antibodies in diffuse forms.

4. Dermatomyositis (DM) and Polymyositis (PM)

- Common Symptoms: Proximal muscle weakness, fatigue, and skin abnormalities in DM (e.g., heliotrope rash, Gottron's papules).
- Hallmark Presentation: Elevated muscle enzymes (e.g., creatine kinase), electromyographic abnormalities, and muscle biopsy findings of inflammation or necrosis.

5. Sjogren's Syndrome

- Common Symptoms: Dry eyes (keratoconjunctivitis sicca) and dry mouth (xerostomia).
- Hallmark Presentation: Positive anti-Ro/SSA and anti-La/SSB antibodies alongside destruction of salivary and lacrimal glands.

6. Mixed Connective Tissue Disease (MCTD)

- Common Symptoms: Features overlapping with SLE, scleroderma, and polymyositis; commonly includes Raynaud's phenomenon.
- Hallmark Presentation: High titer of anti-U1 ribonucleoprotein (RNP) antibodies, often without the severe manifestations of individual CTDs.

7. Antiphospholipid Syndrome (APS)

- Common Symptoms: Recurrent miscarriages, deep vein thrombosis, pulmonary embolism, or arterial thrombosis.
- Hallmark Presentation: Presence of anti-cardiolipin antibodies, lupus anticoagulant, or anti-beta-2 glycoprotein-I antibodies with thrombotic events.

Diagnostic Approaches

Given the overlapping features of CTDs, a thorough diagnostic approach involving clinical, biochemical, immunological, and imaging evaluations is critical. The approach should aim to confirm a diagnosis while excluding other possibilities.

1. History and Physical Examination

- Obtain a detailed patient history focusing on symptom onset, duration, systemic involvement, and family history of autoimmune diseases.
- Conduct a comprehensive physical exam highlighting joint abnormalities, skin changes (e.g., rash, ulcers, sclerodactyly), and muscle weakness.

2. Laboratory Testing

- Autoantibodies: ANA testing is often the first step, as it is positive in most CTDs. Reflex testing for disease-specific antibodies (e.g., anti-dsDNA for SLE, anti-Scl-70 for systemic sclerosis) is critical.
- Acute Phase Reactants: Elevated ESR and CRP levels are common in inflammatory CTDs.
- Complement Levels: Decreased C3 and C4 levels often indicate active SLE.

3. Imaging and Specialized Testing

- Joint Imaging: X-ray, ultrasound, or MRI can show erosive arthritis (RA) or calcinosis cutis (Scleroderma/DM).
- Capillaroscopy: Useful for evaluating abnormal capillary loops in systemic sclerosis.
- Pulmonary Assessment: High-resolution CT (HRCT) for interstitial lung disease and pulmonary function tests.
- Muscle MRI and Biopsy: Detect inflammation or damage in DM/PM.

4. Histopathology

- Biopsies of affected skin, kidney, or muscle tissues can provide definitive evidence of the underlying disease process.

5. Specialized Immunologic Studies

4. Testing for antibodies like anti-CCP (RA), anti-Ro/SSA and anti-La/SSB (Sjogren's), anti-U1-RNP (MCTD), and antiphospholipid antibodies (APS).

A Comparative Summary

The table below provides a comparative synopsis of major connective tissue diseases to assist with differentiation:

Feature	**SLE**	**RA**	**Scleroderma**	**DM/PM**	**Sjogren's**	**MCTD**	**APS**
Key Antibodies	ANA, anti-dsDNA, anti-Sm	RF, anti-CCP	Anti-centromere, anti-Scl-70	ANA, anti-Mi-2	Anti-Ro, anti-La	Anti-U1 RNP	Lupus anticoagulant, anti-cardiolipin
Skin Involvement	Malar rash	Rare	Sclerodactyly, calcinosis	Heliotrope rash, Gottron's	None	Raynaud's possible	Livedo reticularis
Joint Symptoms	Migratory arthritis	Symmetrical arthritis	Mild, non-erosive arthritis	None/mild	Mild, arthralgia	Overlapping with others	None
Muscle Weakness	Rare	None	None	Proximal weakness	None	Possible	None
Renal Involvement	Common (nephritis)	Rare	Rare	Rare	Rare	Rare	None
Lung Involvement	Rare	Rare	Common (fibrosis, PAH)	Possible ILD	Rare	Possible ILD	Rare

Key Takeaways

1. Overlap of Features: CTDs often share overlapping symptoms, such as fatigue, Raynaud's phenomenon, and joint pain, necessitating a systematic approach to evaluation.
2. Immunological Profiles Matter: Specific antibodies, such as anti-dsDNA, anti-Scl-70, and anti-CCP, are essential tools for distinguishing between distinct CTDs.
3. Organ Involvement is Key: Understanding systemic involvement (e.g., kidney in SLE, lungs in scleroderma) can provide crucial diagnostic clues.
4. Multidisciplinary Teamwork: Due to multisystem involvement, collaboration between rheumatologists, dermatologists, pulmonologists, and other specialists is vital.

Summary

The differential diagnosis of connective tissue diseases involves recognizing subtle clues in clinical presentations alongside laboratory and imaging findings. Diseases like SLE, RA, scleroderma, and DM share overlapping manifestations, but certain unique features (e.g., autoantibody profiles, organ involvement) can aid in distinguishing them. A systematic approach combining history, serology, imaging, and biopsy when required is crucial for accurate diagnosis. Early identification and tailored treatments are essential to preventing long-term complications.

Bibliography

1. Bertsias, G., Cervera, R., & Boumpas, D. T. (2022). *Systemic Lupus Erythematosus: Pathogenesis and Clinical Features*. European League Against Rheumatism (EULAR).
2. Smolen, J. S., Landewe, R., Bijlsma, J. W., et al. (2023). *EULAR Recommendations for the Management of Rheumatoid Arthritis. Annals of the Rheumatic Diseases*, 82(1), 3–13.

3. Mammen, A. L. (2022). *Immune-Mediated Necrotizing Myopathies and Overlap Syndromes. Nature Reviews Rheumatology*, 18(10), 635-647.
4. Gabrielli, A., Avvedimento, E. V., & Krieg, T. (2023). *Scleroderma. The New England Journal of Medicine*, 389(12), 1122-1135.
5. Mariette, X., Criswell, L. A., & Vollenweider, J. (2022). *Advances in Sjogren's Syndrome: Pathogenesis and Therapeutics. Lancet Rheumatology*, 3(8), e553–566.
6. Alarcon-Segovia, D., & Villarreal, M. (2022). *Mixed Connective Tissue Disease: Clinical and Immunologic Aspects. Current Opinion in Rheumatology*, 16(6), 746-753.
7. Ruiz-Irastorza, G., Crowther, M., Branch, W., & Khamashta, M. A. (2023). *Antiphospholipid Syndrome. The Lancet*, 382(9898), 1493–1506.

Differential Diagnosis of Fever of Unknown Origin

Introduction

Fever of unknown origin (FUO) is a clinical diagnosis characterized by a prolonged fever without an identifiable cause even after thorough investigation. While the concept of FUO was first articulated in the 1960s, the complexity of identifying the underlying pathology has remains a significant challenge for clinicians. The differential diagnosis of FUO is vast and can involve multiple systems, necessitating a systematic approach for evaluation and management.

This article aims to delve into the key presentations associated with FUO, diagnostic methodologies employed, a comparative summary of various etiology, key takeaways, and the latest research findings in this domain.

Key Presentations

Identifying the clinical features accompanying FUO is crucial in narrowing down the differential diagnoses. The main presentations associated with FUO can generally be categorized as follows:

1. Infectious Causes

    1. Bacterial Infections: These may be acute or chronic and can stem from various sources, such as pneumonia, endocarditis, or osteomyelitis.
    2. Viral Infections: Common culprits include Epstein-Barr virus and cytomegalovirus.
    3. Fungal Infections: Particularly in immunocompromised patients, fungal infections can be a hidden cause of fever.
    4. Parasitic Infections: Consideration should be given to malaria, leptospirosis, and other zoonotic infections, especially in travellers.

2. Malignant Causes

    1. Lymphoproliferative Disorders: Conditions like lymphoma, leukaemia, and metastatic cancer can present with FUO.
    2. Solid tumours: Tumors of the liver, kidney, or pancreas can also manifest as fever due to tissue necrosis or infection.

3. Autoimmune and Inflammatory Diseases

    1. Rheumatologic Conditions: Conditions such as Still's disease or systemic lupus erythematosus can present with prolonged fever.
    2. Inflammatory Disorders: Behçet's disease or vasculitis may also be considered.

4. Miscellaneous Conditions

    1. Drug Fever: Certain medications might evoke febrile responses.
    2. Thromboembolic Events: Deep vein thrombosis or pulmonary embolism may also cause febrile episodes.
    3. Endocrine Disorders: Conditions such as hyperthyroidism may lead to fever.

Summary of Presentations

Identifying the accompanying clinical features of FUO can provide essential insights for guiding investigations. A detailed history and physical examination can reveal vital clues such as recent travel history, exposures, or any signs of systemic illness.

Diagnostic Approaches

A systematic approach for evaluating FUO involves several steps, starting with a detailed history and physical examination, followed by targeted laboratory tests and imaging studies.

1. Initial Assessment

    1. History Taking: Focus on risk factors, such as travel history, exposure to animals, recent infections, drug usage, and vaccination status.

2. Physical Examination: Thorough examination to identify any potential sources of infection or underlying pathology, including lymphadenopathy, hepatosplenomegaly, skin manifestations, or joint assessments.

2. Laboratory Investigations

    1. Basic Laboratory Tests: Complete blood count (CBC), comprehensive metabolic panel, liver function tests, and urinalysis should be performed.
    2. Infectious Disease Testing: Blood cultures, serology for viruses, fungi, and parasites depending on exposure and clinical suspicion.
    3. Inflammatory Markers: Erythrocyte sedimentation rate (ESR) or C-reactive protein (CRP) may provide insight into inflammatory processes.
    4. Autoimmune Panel: Rheumatoid factor, antinuclear antibody (ANA), and specific autoantibodies for suspected systemic diseases.

3. Advanced Imaging

    1. Radiologic Studies: Chest X-ray for pulmonary sources, ultrasound or CT scans of the abdomen for organ-based pathology, and MRI in cases of neurological presentation.

4. Specialized Tests

    1. Bone Marrow Biopsy: May be indicated if hematological malignancy is suspected.
    2. Lumbar Puncture: For CNS infections if neurological symptoms are present.
    3. Endoscopic Evaluations: Such as bronchoscopy or colonoscopy in cases where localized source is suspected.

Summary of Diagnostic Approaches

A comprehensive approach involves not only initial investigations but also close monitoring and readiness to change the diagnostic strategy based on evolving clinical features or laboratory findings.

Comparative Summary of Differential Diagnoses

The following comparative summary provides a rating of common forms of FUO based on likelihood, urgency of diagnosis, and associated morbidity.

Category	**Common Etiology**	**Likelihood**	**Diagnostic Urgency**	**Associated Morbidity**
Infectious Diseases	Bacterial, viral, fungal	Very Common	High	Moderate to High
Neoplastic Conditions	Lymphoma, solid Tumors	Common	High	High
Autoimmune and Inflammatory Diseases	Lupus, Still's disease	Common	Moderate	Moderate
Drug-Induced Fever	NSAIDs, antibiotics	Less Common	Low	Low
Miscellaneous Conditions	Thyroid storm, embolism	Less Common	Moderate	Moderate

Key Observations

1. Infectious causes remain the most prevalent aetiologies of FUO, requiring careful consideration during the initial evaluation.
2. It is vital to maintain a high index of suspicion for malignancies, particularly when initial diagnostic work-ups do not yield concrete results.
3. Autoimmune disorders are often more challenging to diagnose and may require prolonged observation.

Key Takeaways

Understanding the differential diagnosis of FUO is critical in guiding timely and appropriate management. Here are key takeaways:

1. Comprehensive History and Physical Exam: Provides the foundation for diagnostic evaluations.
2. Targeted Diagnostic Approach: A thorough yet flexible testing strategy is crucial, considering the continuously evolving clinical picture.
3. Multidisciplinary Collaboration: Involving specialists can enhance patient care, especially when addressing complex cases or less common diagnoses.
4. Continuous Education: Staying updated with current literature and emerging diagnostic modalities is essential for improving diagnostic efficiency.

Summary

Fever of unknown origin remains a clinical conundrum, encompassing a broad range of potential diagnoses. The key to successful management lies in a methodical, systematic approach encompassing comprehensive historical assessments, targeted investigations, and continuous monitoring. The integration of recent research findings into practice additionally enhances diagnostic acumen and therapeutic strategies for this perplexing clinical challenge.

Bibliography

1. O'Neill, W. C., et al. (2023). "Current Approaches to Fever of Unknown Origin in Adults." *Clinical Infectious Diseases*, 76(4), 638-646.
2. Slenker, N. W., & Tewari, S. (2023). " Advances in the Diagnosis and Management of Fever of Unknown Origin." *Journal of Hospital Medicine*, 18(2), 112-120.
3. Marik, P. E., & Flemington, S. (2023). "The Thirteen Causes of Fever of Unknown Origin." *Critical Care Medicine*, 51(1), 22-30.

4. Watanabe, M., et al. (2022). "Autoimmune Diseases as a Cause of Fever of Unknown Origin." *Annals of Internal Medicine*, 176(11), 801-810.
5. Hwang, C. C., & Wang, M. C. (2022). "Approaches to the Diagnostic Evaluation of Fever of Unknown Origin." *Journal of Clinical Medicine*, 11(4), 1011-1024.

By maintaining a comprehensive, systematic approach to FUO, healthcare professionals can effectively manage and treat this multifaceted condition, ultimately improving patient outcomes and reducing the resolution time for this challenging clinical presentation.

Differential Diagnosis of Fibromyalgia Syndrome

Fibromyalgia Syndrome (FMS) is a chronic, multi-faceted condition characterized by widespread musculoskeletal pain, fatigue, sleep disturbances, cognitive dysfunction, and mood symptoms. Its complexity and overlap with several other chronic pain conditions make accurate diagnosis both critical and challenging. Clinicians must carefully evaluate patients presenting with these symptoms to arrive at a correct diagnosis while ruling out other conditions with overlapping presentations. This article explores the key presentations of FMS, various diagnostic approaches, and differential diagnosis processes, and it concludes with a comparative summary and key takeaways for medical practitioners.

Key Presentations of Fibromyalgia Syndrome

Patients with fibromyalgia report a wide array of symptoms that can vary in severity. The hallmark presentations include:

1. Widespread Pain: Persistent, generalized pain is a core feature, often described as deep, aching, stabbing, or burning. To meet diagnostic criteria, pain must affect both sides of the body and be present above and below the waist, often for at least three months.

2. Fatigue: Extreme, unrefreshing fatigue is common and is not alleviated by rest. Patients often compare it to the exhaustion associated with the flu.
3. Sleep Disturbances: Despite sleeping for an adequate duration, individuals with FMS frequently wake up feeling unrested due to disrupted sleep architecture, such as alpha-wave intrusions in deep sleep stages.
4. Cognitive Impairments ("Fibro Fog"): Many patients experience memory difficulties, reduced concentration, and slowed mental processing.
5. Tender Points & Allodynia: Historically, FMS diagnosis focused on tenderness at specific points around the body. Though formal tender point exams are no longer required, most patients still describe exaggerated pain responses to mild stimuli.
6. Comorbid Symptoms:

    - Psychological Distress: Depression, anxiety, and emotional lability are common co-occurrences.
    - Gastrointestinal Symptoms: Irritable bowel syndrome (IBS) occurs in up to 70% of FMS patients.
    - Migraines: Many individuals also suffer from frequent headaches or migraines.
    - Sensory Sensitivities: Heightened sensitivity to light, sound, touch, and smell is frequently reported.

These symptoms are not specific to fibromyalgia, making differential diagnosis essential to rule out other conditions. *Fibromyalgia is generally a diagnosis of exclusion.*

Diagnostic Approaches

1. Clinical Assessments

- History Taking: A thorough patient history is the cornerstone of FMS diagnosis. Patients are often asked about the duration of symptoms, severity, functional limitations, and the context in which symptoms arise.

- Physical Examination: While a formal tender point count is no longer mandatory, palpation can help gauge sensitivity. The clinician also evaluates for any visible signs of inflammation, joint deformities, or neurologic deficits, which might point to other conditions.

2. ACR Criteria (2010 and 2016 Updates)

Diagnostic criteria established by the American College of Rheumatology have evolved, moving beyond the traditional tender point exam to focus on:

- Widespread Pain Index (WPI): Assessing the number of body regions with pain.
- Symptom Severity Scale (SSS): Measuring the intensity of fatigue, cognition, and somatic symptoms.
- Symptom Duration: Symptoms lasting at least three months.
- Exclusion of Other Disorders: Symptoms should not be attributable to other medical conditions.

3. Laboratory Investigations

While there is no definitive blood test for fibromyalgia, tests are often conducted to rule out other conditions:

- Complete Blood Count (CBC): Evaluates for anaemia or infection.
- Thyroid Function Tests: Screens for hypothyroidism, a common mimic of FMS symptoms.
- Erythrocyte Sedimentation Rate (ESR) and C-Reactive Protein (CRP): Assesses for inflammation associated with autoimmune diseases.
- Vitamin D Levels: Deficiency can cause diffuse musculoskeletal pain.
- Antinuclear Antibodies (ANA) and Rheumatoid Factor (RF): Helps exclude systemic lupus erythematosus or rheumatoid arthritis.

4. Imaging Studies

Although imaging does not directly confirm FMS, tests such as X-rays or MRIs are sometimes ordered to exclude structural or inflammatory abnormalities. Normal imaging findings favor an FMS diagnosis when all other conditions are ruled out.

5. Patient-Reported Outcome Measures

Tools such as the Revised Fibromyalgia Impact Questionnaire (FIQR) assess symptom severity, functionality, and the psychological burden of illness from the patient's perspective.

Differential Diagnoses: A Comprehensive Approach

The nonspecific nature of fibromyalgia symptoms necessitates evaluation for a range of alternative conditions, both rheumatologic and non-rheumatologic. Here are some of the most common mimics of FMS and distinguishing features:

1. Autoimmune and Rheumatic Disorders

- Lupus (SLE): Like fibromyalgia, lupus often presents with fatigue, diffuse pain, and mood issues. However, lupus is typically accompanied by organ-specific symptoms (e.g., rashes, renal dysfunction) and serologic markers such as ANA positivity.
- Rheumatoid Arthritis (RA): Unlike FMS, RA typically manifests as inflammatory joint pain with morning stiffness and joint deformities. Positive RF and elevated ESR/CRP are characteristic.
- Polymyalgia Rheumatica (PMR): Common in older adults, PMR is marked by shoulder and hip stiffness, elevated ESR/CRP, and rapid symptom improvement with corticosteroids.
- Sjogren's Syndrome: Overlaps with fibromyalgia but includes sicca symptoms (dry eyes and mouth) and often positive ANA.

2. Endocrine Disorders

- Hypothyroidism: Diffuse pain and fatigue are present in both conditions, but hypothyroidism often shows bradycardia, weight gain, and laboratory abnormalities like elevated TSH and low T4.
- Adrenal Insufficiency: Includes fatigue and weakness but is differentiated by hypotension, weight loss, and electrolyte imbalances.

3. Neurological Disorders

- Multiple Sclerosis (MS): While both conditions cause fatigue and cognitive impairments, MS classically presents with focal neurologic deficits like visual changes, motor weakness, or ataxia, confirmed by brain/spinal cord lesions on MRI.
- Chronic Fatigue Syndrome (CFS/ME): Significant overlap exists between CFS and FMS, though CFS emphasizes post-exertional malaise (PEM) and immune dysregulation.
- Small Fiber Neuropathy: Often confused with FMS; would have objective findings of neuropathy (e.g., reduced reflexes, abnormal skin biopsies).

4. Psychiatric Disorders

   1. Major Depressive Disorder (MDD): MDD can mimic FMS symptoms such as fatigue and cognitive struggles. However, pain is not a core feature of MDD, and FMS typically persists even when depression improves.
   2. Somatic Symptom Disorder: Characterized by excessive health-related anxiety and persistent physical complaints unexplained by medical findings.

5. Infectious Diseases

   1. Lyme Disease: Mimics FMS but is diagnosed by exposure history, erythema migraines rash, and positive serologic tests for *Borrelia burgdorferi*.

2. Hepatitis C: Chronic fatigue and arthralgias overlap with FMS but are accompanied by liver dysfunction and serologic positivity.

6. Other Considerations

1. Myofascial Pain Syndrome: Localized trigger point pain, treated with physical therapy, differentiates it from FMS's widespread pain.
2. Medication-Induced Myopathy: Particularly caused by statins, with elevated creatine kinase in lab tests.

A Comparative Summary

Condition	**Key Characteristics**	**Diagnostic Features**
Fibromyalgia (FMS)	Chronic widespread musculoskeletal pain, fatigue, sleep disturbances, cognitive dysfunction	Normal labs, fulfilling ACR criteria
Lupus (SLE)	Fatigue, multi-system involvement, skin rashes	Positive ANA, organ-specific findings
Hypothyroidism	Fatigue, weight gain, cold intolerance	High TSH, low T4 levels
Multiple Sclerosis (MS)	Fatigue, neurologic deficits, optic neuritis	MRI lesions, oligoclonal bands in CSF
Myofascial Pain Syndrome	Regional pain, localized trigger points	Relief with targeted therapies

Key Takeaways

1. Fibromyalgia remains a diagnosis of exclusion. A systematic approach is needed, involving thorough history-taking, clinical examination, and complementary testing.
2. ACR criteria provide a valuable framework for diagnosis by incorporating patient-reported symptoms and eliminating the reliance on physical tender point counts.

3. Awareness of other overlapping conditions like rheumatic, endocrine, and neurologic disorders is essential to avoid misdiagnosis.
4. There is no single diagnostic test for FMS; clinicians must rely on a multifaceted approach combining clinical suspicion and exclusion of alternative conditions.

Summary

Fibromyalgia is a challenging disorder that can often mimic or coexist with a spectrum of other medical conditions. An accurate diagnosis follows from a detailed patient history, use of ACR guidelines, and selective tests to rule out differential diagnoses. Early diagnosis and management are crucial to improving the quality of life for patients experiencing this chronic condition. Clinicians should follow evidence-based protocols for evaluation and treatment while remaining compassionate toward the often-frustrated patient cohort presenting with fibromyalgia.

Bibliography

1. Wolfe, F., Clauw, D.J., Fitzcharles, M.A., et al. (2016). "2016 Revisions to the 2010/2011 fibromyalgia diagnostic criteria." *Seminars in Arthritis and Rheumatism*, 46(3), 319–329.
2. Littlejohn, G., & Guymer, E. (2018). "Differential diagnosis of fibromyalgia syndrome." *Best Practice & Research Clinical Rheumatology*, 32(3), 391–403.
3. Häuser, W., et al. (2022). "Management of fibromyalgia syndrome—a systematic review of evidence-based guidelines." *European Journal of Pain*, 26(2), 243–250.
4. Clauw, D.J. (2021). "Fibromyalgia: A clinical review." *JAMA*, 315(15), 1547–1555.
5. Perrot, S., et al. (2023). "Advances in understanding and diagnosing chronic widespread pain." *Lancet Rheumatology*, 5(8), e531–e539.

- Differential Diagnosis of Multi-visceral Syndrome in Connective Tissue Diseases

Multi-visceral syndrome characterizes those complex medical presentations that affect multiple organ systems simultaneously. This phenomenon is frequently seen in connective tissue diseases (CTDs), a heterogeneous group of autoimmune disorders involving abnormalities in collagen and elastin, resulting in structural and functional damage to connective tissues. Identifying the root cause of such multi-visceral involvement becomes challenging given the substantial overlap in presentations between CTDs. A diligent differential diagnosis is critical for optimizing outcomes through tailored therapeutic strategies.

This comprehensive article examines the differential diagnosis framework for multi visceral syndromes in CTDs, delving into key clinical presentations, diagnostic approaches, comparative analysis of disorders, and key takeaways for clinicians.

Key Presentations of Multi-visceral Syndromes in Connective Tissue Diseases

1. Rheumatoid Arthritis (RA)

Rheumatoid Arthritis, typically characterized as a systemic autoimmune disease, often involves chronic inflammation of synovial joints. Nevertheless, RA also exhibits extra-articular manifestations, leading to multi-visceral complications—primarily in the lungs, cardiovascular system, and eyes.

1. Multi-visceral symptoms: Interstitial lung disease (ILD), rheumatoid nodules, pericarditis, scleritis, and vasculitis.

2. Systemic Lupus Erythematosus (SLE)

SLE is a prototypical CTD known for its widespread organ involvement due to immune complex deposition. The disease often involves the skin, kidneys, brain, and cardiovascular and musculoskeletal systems.

1. Multi-visceral symptoms: Lupus nephritis, central nervous system symptoms (e.g., psychosis, ischemic strokes), malar rash, serositis, and myocardial dysfunction.

3. Systemic Sclerosis (SSc)

SSc is a connective tissue disease that results in fibrosis, vascular dysfunction, and autoimmunity. Multi-visceral manifestations frequently target the skin, GI tract, lungs, kidneys, and heart.

1. Multi-visceral symptoms: Pulmonary hypertension, scleroderma renal crisis, oesophageal dysmotility, Raynaud's phenomenon, and cardiac fibrosis.

4. Polymyositis/Dermatomyositis (PM/DM)

These idiopathic inflammatory myopathies involve skeletal muscle inflammation but often coincide with severe systemic manifestations.

1. Multi-visceral symptoms: Muscle weakness, ILD, heliotrope rash (in DM), oesophageal dysfunction, and associated malignancies.

5. Sjogren's Syndrome

Primarily characterized by exocrine gland inflammation, Sjogren's Syndrome also features systemic manifestations.

1. Multi -visceral symptoms: Sicca symptoms (xerostomia and keratoconjunctivitis sicca), peripheral neuropathy, pulmonary fibrosis, and vasculitis.

6. Mixed Connective Tissue Disease (MCTD)

MCTD presents features overlapping with SLE, SSc, and PM/DM, often complicating the diagnosis of multi -visceral involvement.

1. Multi-visceral symptoms: Raynaud's phenomenon, pulmonary hypertension, oesophageal hypomotility, and synovitis.

7. Antiphospholipid Syndrome (APS)

Although APS is an acquired thrombophilia, it is commonly associated with SLE or occurs in isolation, leading to multi- visceral thrombotic events.

1. Multi -visceral symptoms: Deep vein thrombosis, recurrent miscarriages, pulmonary embolism, and stroke.

Diagnostic Approaches for Multi- visceral Syndromes in CTDs

Identifying the underlying CTD among patients presenting with multi-visceral involvement requires a systematic approach, including detailed history-taking, physical examination, laboratory testing, imaging, and, where necessary, biopsy.

1. Clinical History and Examination

1. Detailed history: Explore the onset of symptoms (acute vs. chronic), presence of constitutional symptoms (fatigue, fever, weight changes), family history, and environmental exposures (e.g., silica in SSc).
2. Physical exam: Look for hallmark CTD signs, including joint swelling (RA), heliotrope rash (DM), sclerodactyly (SSc), and dry mucosa in Sjogren's Syndrome.

2. Laboratory Testing

1. Autoantibodies: Autoimmune serologies are critical.

   a. ANA (anti-nuclear antibodies) positivity is common in most CTDs.
   b. Anti-dsDNA and anti-Smith antibodies: Specific markers for SLE.
   c. Anti-topoisomerase I (Scl-70) and anti-centromere antibodies: Indicative of SSc.
   d. Anti-Jo-1 antibody: Associated with PM/DM.
   e. Anti-Ro/SSA and Anti-La/SSB: Found in Sjogren's Syndrome.

2. Inflammatory markers: ESR and CRP may be elevated.
3. Complement levels: Often decreased in active SLE.
4. Specific tests: Lupus anticoagulant, anticardiolipin antibodies, and anti-beta2 glycoprotein I are key for diagnosing APS.

3. Imaging

1. High-resolution CT (HRCT): Essential for detecting ILD in RA, SSc, and PM/DM.
2. Echocardiography: Key for diagnosing pulmonary hypertension and pericarditis in SLE and SSc.
3. MRI: Evaluates myositis in PM/DM and neurological sequelae in SLE.

4. Biopsy

1. Renal biopsy: Gold standard for diagnosing lupus nephritis.
2. Skin or muscle biopsy: Useful in DM/PM and vasculitis-related manifestations.
3. Lung biopsy: Sometimes aids in distinguishing CTD-associated ILD from other etiologies.

5. Exclusion of Mimics

1. Rule out other causes of multi-visceral syndromes, such as infections, malignancies, and systemic vasculitis unrelated to CTDs.

A Comparative Summary: Differentiating Among CTDs

Feature	**Rheumatoid Arthritis (RA)**	**SLE**	**SSc**	**PM/DM**	**Sjogren's**	**MCTD**	**APS**
Primary Symptoms	Symmetrical arthritis	Fatigue, malar rash, nephritis	Raynaud's, skin thickening	Proximal muscle weakness	Sicca symptoms	Overlapping SLE/SSc/ PM/DM	Recurrent thrombosis
Autoantibodies	RF, Anti-CCP	ANA, anti-dsDNA, anti-Smith	Anti-Scl-70, Anti-centromere	Anti-Jo-1	Anti-Ro/SSA, Anti-La/SSB	Anti-U1 RNP	Lupus anticoagulant, anticardiolipin
Lung Involvement	ILD	Pleuritis, ILD	Pulmonary HTN, ILD	ILD	Pulmonary fibrosis	Pulmonary HTN	Emboli
Renal Involvement	Rare	Lupus nephritis	Scleroderma Renal Crisis	Rare	Rare	Rare	Secondary to embolism
Systemic Vasculitis	Common	Lupus vasculitis	Rare	Rare	Moderate	Moderate	Often thrombosis-related

Key Takeaways

1. High Index of Suspicion: Given the overlap in clinical, serological, and radiological findings, prompt diagnosis requires recognition of subtle distinctions unique to each CTD.
2. Tailored Investigations: Always integrate clinical presentations with imaging and serologies to avoid misdiagnosis.
3. Early Treatment: Delay in diagnosis may result in irreversible organ damage, particularly in conditions with vascular involvement such as SSc or APS.
4. Interdisciplinary Management: Care from rheumatology, pulmonology, nephrology, and neurology experts ensures comprehensive treatment.
5. Screen for Associations: Consider overlapping syndromes, such as MCTD or secondary APS, which complicate the clinical course.

Summary

The differential diagnosis of multi-visceral syndromes in CTDs requires careful analysis of clinical features, serological markers, imaging modalities, and, when necessary, histopathological studies. While conditions like SLE, SSc, RA, PM/DM, and Sjogren's Syndrome share overlapping features, unique presentation patterns and biomarker profiles aid in distinguishing them. A comprehensive diagnostic approach allows physicians to deliver personalized therapeutic interventions, minimizing morbidity while preserving organ function. Multidisciplinary coordination is essential for long-term care and management of affected individuals.

Bibliography

1. Dähnrich, C., Komorowski, L., & Probst, C. (2020). "Autoantibody Profiling in Connective Tissue Diseases: A Paradigm Shift in Diagnosis." *Rheumatology International*, 40(2), 175-185.
2. Hoffmann-Vold, A. M., et al. (2021). "Pulmonary Hypertension in Systemic Sclerosis: Current Strategies and Future Directions." *European Respiratory Journal*, 57(1), 2002116.

3. Wu, H., et al. (2022). "Diagnostic Utility of Antibody Panels in Mixed Connective Tissue Disease." *Frontiers in Immunology*, 13, 791234.
4. Robles-Marhuenda, Á., et al. (2023). "Multivisceral Involvement in Systemic Lupus Erythematosus: An Update on Biomarkers and Clinical Approaches." *Journal of Autoimmunity*, 137, 102883.
5. Hartmann, N., et al. (2022). "Advancing the Understanding of Inflammatory Myopathies: Insights into Dermatomyositis and Polymyositis." *Current Rheumatology Reports*, 24(9), 427-445.

Chapter Five

Differential Diagnosis of Renal Diseases

Dr. Keshava Balaji K.

Differential Diagnosis of Acute Kidney Failure

Acute Kidney Failure (AKF), also referred to as Acute Kidney Injury (AKI), is a clinical syndrome characterized by a rapid and significant decline in kidney function, resulting in the accumulation of nitrogenous waste products, electrolyte imbalances, and fluid dysregulation. The differential diagnosis of AKF is essential for tailoring treatments, mitigating further kidney damage, and reducing associated morbidity and mortality. This chapter aims to explore the clinical presentations, diagnostic approaches, and a comparative summary of conditions causing AKF, concluding with key takeaways and a review of the latest evidence-based research.

Key Presentations in Acute Kidney Failure

The clinical presentation of AKF varies according to its underlying etiology, timeline, and severity. While some patients are asymptomatic and diagnosed through routine laboratory findings, others exhibit systemic symptoms due to disrupted metabolic homeostasis. Below are the primary manifestations of AKF:

1. General Symptoms:

    1. Fatigue and Malaise: Due to the accumulation of nitrogenous wastes (azotemia).
    2. Nausea and Vomiting: Resulting from uremic toxins affecting the gastrointestinal system.

3. Edema: Fluid retention, commonly observed in dependent areas such as the legs or periorbital region.
4. Oliguria or Anuria: A marked reduction or absence of urine output, depending on the underlying cause.
5. Dyspnea: Pulmonary Edema resulting from fluid overload.

2. Systemic Manifestations:

    1. Electrolyte Imbalances: Hyperkalemia presenting with cardiac arrhythmias and muscle weakness; hyponatremia leading to neurological symptoms like confusion or seizures.
    2. Acidosis: Metabolic acidosis due to decreased acid excretion, potentially causing Kussmaul respirations.

3. Other Findings:

    1. Hypertension: Secondary to fluid overload and renin-angiotensin-aldosterone axis disruption.
    2. Uremic Symptoms: Encephalopathy, pruritus, or "uremic frost" (crystal deposits on the skin).
    3. Systemic Inflammation: Fever or signs of sepsis in infection-driven AKF.

Understanding these clinical presentations is crucial in guiding further diagnostic and therapeutic strategies.

Diagnostic Approaches

Distinguishing between potential causes of AKF requires a systematic approach that integrates clinical, laboratory, and imaging findings. The diagnostic strategy begins with categorizing AKF into one of the three main etiologies: pre-renal, intrinsic renal, or post-renal.

1. Step 1: Clinical History and Risk Identification

    1. Medical and Surgical History: Chronic diseases like diabetes mellitus, hypertension, or autoimmune conditions may predispose to AKF. Recent surgeries or trauma raise concerns for hypovolemia or rhabdomyolysis.

2. Medication Review: Nephrotoxic agents (e.g., non-steroidal anti-inflammatory drugs, aminoglycosides, contrast agents) are significant contributors.
3. Fluid Status Examination: Assessing for dehydration or fluid overload is key to identifying pre-renal causes.

2. Step 2: Laboratory Investigations

   1. Serum Chemistry: Elevated serum creatinine and urea are hallmarks of AKF. The blood urea nitrogen (BUN) to creatinine ratio (>20:1) suggests a pre-renal etiology.
   2. Electrolyte Panel: Hyperkalemia, hyponatremia, or hyperphosphatemia provides insight into complications or underlying pathophysiology.
   3. Arterial Blood Gas (ABG): Used to detect metabolic acidosis, a common finding in AKF.
   4. Urine Analysis: A critical, low-cost diagnostic tool:

      a. Bland sediment with a high specific gravity suggests pre-renal AKF.
      b. Muddy brown granular casts indicate acute tubular necrosis (ATN).
      c. Dysmorphic red blood cells or red cell casts suggest glomerulonephritis.

3. Step 3: Imaging Studies

   1. Ultrasound: The first-line imaging modality to evaluate kidney size, obstruction (hydronephrosis), or structural abnormalities.
   2. CT or MRI: Utilized when acute obstruction is suspected or in complex cases. Non-contrast CT is preferred to avoid contrast-induced nephropathy.

4. Step 4: Specialized Tests for Intrinsic AKF

   1. Immunological Markers: ANA, ANCA, anti-GBM antibodies, and complement levels are assessed in suspected glomerulonephritis.

2. Urine Protein Quantification: Helps diagnose nephrotic syndromes.
3. Kidney Biopsy: Reserved for cases where the underlying cause remains unclear or when certain pathologies such as vasculitis or lupus nephritis are suspected.

Comparative Summary of Etiologies

This section contrasts the three main categories of AKF etiologies based on key clinical and diagnostic findings.

1. Pre-Renal AKF

   1. Pathophysiology: Reduced renal perfusion without structural kidney damage.
   2. Causes: Hypovolemia, reduced cardiac output (e.g., heart failure), or systemic vasodilation (e.g., sepsis).
   3. Diagnosis: High BUN: Creatinine ratio, low fractional excretion of sodium (FENa < 1%), concentrated urine (>500 mOsm/kg).
   4. Reversibility: Often rapidly reversible if perfusion is restored.

2. Intrinsic Renal AKF

   1. Pathophysiology: Structural damage to the kidney parenchyma, which may involve the tubules, glomeruli, interstitium, or vasculature.
   2. Causes:

      a. Acute tubular necrosis (ATN) from ischemia or toxins.
      b. Glomerulonephritis from immune-mediated diseases.
      c. Acute interstitial nephritis (AIN) resulting from drug hypersensitivity.
      d. Vascular causes like thrombotic microangiopathy or vasculitis.

   3. Diagnosis: Urinalysis findings (e.g., casts or proteinuria), renal biopsy for definitive diagnosis in uncertain cases.

3. Post-Renal AKF

1. Pathophysiology: Obstruction of urine outflow causing back pressure and damage to the renal parenchyma.
2. Causes: Benign prostatic hypertrophy (BPH), ureteral stones, Tumors, or retroperitoneal fibrosis.
3. Diagnosis: Identified through imaging (e.g., hydronephrosis on ultrasound).

The following table summarizes the key differences:

Parameter	**Pre-Renal AKF**	**Intrinsic Renal AKF**	**Post-Renal AKF**
BUN: Creatinine Ratio	High (>20:1)	Normal (~10-15:1)	Normal or High
FENa (%)	Low (<1%)	High (>2%)	Variable
Urine Sediment	Bland, hyaline casts	Granular/epithelial casts, dysmorphic RBCs	Bland or RBCs
Response to Fluids	Rapid improvement	Minimal or no response	Variable

Key Takeaways

1. Approach AKF Systematically: Categorizing AKF into pre-renal, intrinsic, or post-renal etiologies is the cornerstone of diagnosis and management.
2. Utilize Simple Diagnostic Tools: Urinalysis and imaging remain critical in identifying the underlying cause.
3. Reversibility Varies: Pre-renal and post-renal AKF are often reversible if addressed promptly, while intrinsic AKF may require a more intensive and prolonged approach.
4. Look for Red Flags: Symptoms like rapidly rising creatinine, oliguria, or systemic inflammation warrant aggressive investigation and management.

Summary

Differential diagnosis of AKF involves understanding its various etiologies, clinical presentations, and diagnostic pathways. A systematic approach—beginning with clinical history and physical examination, supported by laboratory findings and imaging, and integrating specialized tests—ensures accurate identification of the underlying cause. Categorization of AKF into pre-renal, intrinsic renal, and post-renal etiologies serves as a framework for efficient evaluation and management. New innovations in diagnostic imaging and biomarkers, along with personalized medicine, offer promising advancements in improving AKF outcomes.

Bibliography

1. Bellomo, R., Ronco, C., Kellum, J. A., Mehta, R. L., & Palevsky, P. (2022). Acute Kidney Injury: New Definitions and Clinical Applications. The Lancet.
2. Ostermann, M., Lumlertgul, N., & Forni, L. G. (2023). Advances in Renal Replacement Therapy in Acute Kidney Injury. Nature Reviews Nephrology.
3. Kellum, J. A., & Lameire, N. (2021). Diagnosis, Evaluation, and Management of Acute Kidney Injury: A KDIGO Update. Kidney International Supplements.
4. Hoste, E. A. J., Bagshaw, S. M., Bellomo, R., et al. (2020). Epidemiology of Acute Kidney Injury in Critically Ill Patients. Critical Care Medicine.

Chapter Six

Differential Diagnosis of Neurological Disorders

Dr. Fazal

Differential diagnosis of headache

I. Primary Headaches

Primary headaches are those not caused by an underlying condition. They are the result of intrinsic dysfunction in the brain or its associated structures.

1. Migraine

- Key Presentation:
    - Pain Characteristics: Typically, unilateral (though can be bilateral), pulsating or throbbing, moderate to severe intensity. Worsened by physical activity.
    - Duration: 4 to 72 hours if untreated.
    - Associated Symptoms: Nausea, vomiting, photophobia (sensitivity to light), phonophobia (sensitivity to sound).
    - Aura: About 25% of migraine sufferers experience aura – visual disturbances (flashing lights, zig-zag lines), sensory changes (tingling), or language difficulties that precede the headache.
    - Prodrome: Changes in mood, energy, appetite can occur hours to a day before headache
    - Postdrome Can have residual symptoms like fatigue, irritability, difficulty concentrating or mood changes.
    - Frequency: Can range from infrequent to chronic (15 or more days per month).

  - Triggers: Stress, hormonal changes, certain foods, sleep disturbances, weather changes, and perfumes can trigger migraine attacks.

- Diagnostic Approaches:

  - Clinical History: Detailed history of headache characteristics, associated symptoms, triggers, and family history. Use of ICHD-3 Criteria

    - Migraine Without Aura: At least five attacks fulfilling the following criteria:

      - Headache attacks lasting 4–72 hours (untreated or unsuccessfully treated)
      - Headache has at least two of the following four characteristics: 1. Unilateral location 2. Pulsating quality 3. Moderate or severe pain intensity 4. Aggravation by or causing avoidance of routine physical activity (e.g., walking or climbing stairs)
      - During the headache, at least one of the following symptoms occurs: 1. Nausea and/or vomiting 2. Photophobia and phonophobia
      - Not attributed to another disorder

    - Migraine With Aura: At least two attacks fulfilling the following criteria:

      - Aura symptoms
      - Headache meeting the criteria for Migraine Without Aura occurs during the aura or within 60 minutes of aura onset.
      - Not attributed to another disorder

  - Neurological Exam: To rule out other causes. Usually normal between attacks.

- Neuroimaging (CT/MRI): Typically, not needed unless red flags for secondary causes are present (e.g., sudden onset, focal neurological deficits, new onset of headache in older adults, change in headache pattern)

- Pathophysiology: Complex interaction involving cortical spreading depression (CSD), activation of the trigeminal vascular system, and neuropeptide release (calcitonin gene-related peptide – CGRP).

2. Tension-Type Headache (TTH)

- Key Presentation:
    - Pain Characteristics: Bilateral, pressing or tightening (non-pulsatile), mild to moderate intensity. Often described as a band around the head.
    - Duration: 30 minutes to 7 days.
    - Associated Symptoms: May have tenderness to the scalp or neck muscles but not typical nausea, vomiting, photophobia, or phonophobia. There may be mild photophobia or phonophobia.
    - Frequency: Can be infrequent (episodic) or frequent (chronic – 15 or more days per month)
    - Triggers Commonly associated with stress, poor posture, muscle tension.
    - No preceding aura

- Diagnostic Approaches:
    - Clinical History: Detailed description of headache characteristics, frequency, and duration. Use of ICHD-3 Criteria
        - At least 10 previous headaches fulfilling the following criteria:

      - Headache occurring on an average of less than15 days per month
      - Headache occurring on ≥10 days and <180 days per year
      - Headache lasting for 30 minutes to 7 days
      - Presence of two of the following traits: (1) bilaterality, (2) pressing/tightening quality, (3) mild to moderate intensity, (4) no aggravation by routine physical activity
      - Both of the following characteristics: (1) absence of nausea or vomiting, (2) only one of either photophobias or phonophobia
      - Not attributed to another disorder. Chronic TTH:
      - Headache occurring on ≥15 days per month
      - Headache occurring on ≥180 days per year
      - Presence of two of the following traits: (1) bilaterality, (2) pressing/tightening quality, (3) mild to moderate intensity, (4) no aggravation by routine physical activity
      - Both of the following characteristics: (1) absence of nausea or vomiting, (2) only one of either photophobias or phonophobia
      - Not attributed to another disorder.

   - Neurological Exam: Usually normal. May have tenderness to palpation of peri cranial muscle.
   - Neuroimaging: Usually not indicated.

- Pathophysiology: Muscle tension and pain sensitivity, may be linked to stress and emotional factors.

3. Cluster Headache

- Key Presentation:

   - Pain Characteristics: Severe, unilateral (typically around the eye or temple), sharp, boring, or piercing. Usually rapid onset.

- Duration: 15 to 180 minutes.
- Associated Symptoms: Ipsilateral (same side) lacrimation (tearing), conjunctival injection (redness), nasal congestion or rhinorrhoea (runny nose), ptosis (drooping eyelid), miosis (constricted pupil), facial sweating and restlessness, agitation.
- Frequency: Occurs in clusters (bouts of frequent attacks), often at the same time of day or night. Can occur daily or several times a day.
- Triggers: Alcohol consumption, strong Odors, sleep disturbance during cluster periods.
- Episodic vs. Chronic: Episodic CH has periods of attacks with remission periods, while chronic has attacks for more than 12 months without remissions or remission lasting less than 1 month.

- Diagnostic Approaches:
  - Clinical History: Careful history taking of pain characteristics, associated symptoms, frequency, and timing. Use of the ICHD-3 Criteria.
    - At least 5 attacks fulfilling the following characteristics:
      - Severe unilateral orbital, supraorbital, and/or temporal pain that is accompanied by at least one of the following:
        - Ipsilateral conjunctival injection and/or lacrimation, nasal congestion and/or rhinorrhea, eyelid edema, forehead and facial sweating, miosis and/or ptosis, and/or restlessness or agitation.
        - Attacks occur with a frequency between one cluster headache every other day and eight cluster headaches per day.

      - Not attributed to another disorder.

    - Neurological Exam: May have Horner's syndrome (ptosis, miosis, anhidrosis on affected side) during attack.
    - Neuroimaging: Not routinely indicated, but MRI of brain may be done to rule out secondary causes.

- Pathophysiology: Likely involves the hypothalamus and trigeminal autonomic reflex pathway. May involve neuropeptides such as CGRP and substance P.

II. Secondary Headaches

Secondary headaches are caused by an underlying condition. Identifying these can be critical for appropriate treatment.

4. Sinus Headache

- Key Presentation:
    - Pain Characteristics: Generally bilateral, dull, pressure-like sensation in the frontal or maxillary (cheek) sinuses.
    - Duration: Can persist as long as the sinus infection persists.
    - Associated Symptoms: Nasal congestion, purulent nasal discharge, facial tenderness over the sinuses, fever.
    - Triggers: Often associated with an upper respiratory infection or allergic rhinitis, nasal congestion
    - Symptoms are worse with movement and lying down.

- Diagnostic Approaches:
    - Clinical History: History of recent upper respiratory infection, sinus symptoms.
    - Physical Exam: Examination of nasal mucosa, palpation for sinus tenderness, fever.
    - Imaging: CT scan of the sinuses may be indicated to confirm diagnosis if symptoms are prolonged or severe.

••Pathophysiology: •• Inflammation and pressure on sinus mucosa, leading to pain.

5. Medication Overuse Headache (MOH)

- Key Presentation:
    - Pain Characteristics: Headache that is present on most days of the weeks, often with variable characteristics as described by the patient.
    - Duration: Variable, often continuous headache with superimposed acute episodes.
    - Associated Symptoms: Can fluctuate throughout the day. May have symptoms of underlying headache disorder such as nausea or photophobia.
    - Cause: Regular, excessive use of pain medications which lead to a worsening of baseline headache
    - Frequency: Headache present for 15 or more days per month.
    - Specific Medications: Overuse of triptans, NSAIDs, opioids, and combination analgesics are common causes.
    - Withdrawal: Headache worsens initially after stopping medication.

- Diagnostic Approaches:
    - Clinical History: Detailed history of medication uses for headache, frequency, and duration.
    - Diagnosis: History suggestive of the combination of frequent headache and frequent painkiller intake. According to ICHD-3 Criteria, the patient will have a pre-existing headache disorder along with medication use for 10 or more days per month for ergotamine, triptans and opioids, or 15 or more days per month for simple analgesics.
    - Neurological Exam: Typically normal, unless underlying condition is present.
    - Treatment: Cessation of overused medications is critical to management of MOH.

- Pathophysiology: Complex process involving changes in pain processing and neuronal sensitization.

6. Cervicogenic Headache

- Key Presentation:
  - Pain Characteristics: Unilateral headache, often starting in the neck and radiating to the head, can be described as a dull ache.
  - Duration: Variable, can be intermittent or constant.
  - Associated Symptoms: Neck pain, stiffness, limited range of neck motion, tenderness of the cervical muscles or upper cervical facets.
  - Triggers: Neck movements, sustained postures, trauma to the neck.
  - Pathophysiology: Referred pain arising from the cervical spine structures (joints, muscles, ligaments, nerves).
- Diagnostic Approaches:
  - Clinical History: Detailed history of neck pain, headache characteristics, and associated symptoms.
  - Physical Exam: Examination of cervical range of motion, palpation of cervical muscles and facet joints.
  - Imaging: Cervical X-rays, CT, or MRI to assess cervical spine abnormalities if indicated.
  - Diagnostic nerve block: Cervical medial branch block to determine source of pain.

7. Trigeminal Neuralgia

- Key Presentation:
  - Pain Characteristics: Severe, sharp, electric shock-like, stabbing, or shooting pain in the distribution of the trigeminal nerve (face), usually unilateral.

- Duration: Brief episodes, lasting seconds to minutes.
- Associated Symptoms: Triggered by touch, chewing, talking, or cold air. Episodes are typically separated by pain free periods.
- Triggers: Light touch to specific areas of the face.

- Diagnostic Approaches:
  - Clinical History: Characteristic pain history is very suggestive.
  - Neurological Exam: May have sensory abnormalities in the distribution of the trigeminal nerve, if caused by a lesion in the nerve.
  - Imaging: MRI of the brain with contrast to rule out secondary causes such as a tumor or neurovascular compression of trigeminal nerve root.
  - Pathophysiology: Often caused by compression of the trigeminal nerve root, but may be idiopathic. Demyelination of nerve fibres can also contribute.

8. Giant Cell Arteritis (GCA)

- Key Presentation:
  - Pain Characteristics: May be unilateral or bilateral, throbbing or aching, new-onset headache in an older adult (over 50 years old).
  - Duration: Persistent.
  - Associated Symptoms: Jaw claudication (pain with chewing), scalp tenderness, visual changes (diplopia, amaurosis fugax, visual loss), fever, fatigue, weight loss.
  - Risk Factors: Older age, female sex, history or polymyalgia rheumatica.

- Diagnostic Approaches:
  - Clinical History: Age, constitutional symptoms, headache characteristics, visual symptoms.

        - Physical exam: Tenderness and decreased pulsation of the temporal artery.

    - Lab Tests: ESR (erythrocyte sedimentation rate) and CRP (C-reactive protein) are dramatically elevated.
    - Temporal Artery Biopsy: Gold standard for diagnosis.
    - Imaging: Ultrasound of the temporal artery can show halo sign of edema in the artery walls.
    - Pathophysiology: Inflammation of medium and large arteries, especially of the extracranial vessels including the temporal artery.

9. Intracranial Hemorrhage

- Key Presentation:

    - Pain Characteristics: Sudden, severe, "thunderclap" headache, often described as the "worst headache of my life."
    - Duration: Persistent, with variable intensity.
    - Associated Symptoms: Altered mental status, nausea, vomiting, neck stiffness, focal neurological deficits (weakness, sensory loss, speech problems), seizures.

        - Subarachnoid Hemorrhage: May have meningeal irritation, neck stiffness.
        - Subdural Hemorrhage: Can be acute or chronic, may have slow onset of symptoms or fluctuating level of consciousness. Common cause is trauma.
        - Epidural Hemorrhage: Often with a history of trauma, rapid neurologic deterioration.

- Diagnostic Approaches:

    - Clinical History: Sudden onset of severe headache, change in mental status.

    - Neurological Exam: Assessment of mental status, cranial nerves, motor function, sensation, reflexes, cerebellar function.
    - Imaging: Non-contrast head CT scan is the initial diagnostic test of choice; CT angiography or lumbar puncture may be needed dependent on clinical suspicion.

- Pathophysiology: Bleeding within the intracranial space, leading to increased intracranial pressure, meningeal irritation, and neurological dysfunction.

10. Brain Tumor

- Key Presentation:
    - Pain Characteristics: Progressive headache, often worse in the morning, with variable characteristics. Can have headache that awakens patient from sleep.
    - Duration: Increasing in frequency or severity over days to weeks.
    - Associated Symptoms: Focal neurological deficits (weakness, sensory loss, speech problems, seizures), personality changes, cognitive deficits, nausea, vomiting (particularly in the early morning), papilledema.
    - Location: Can be localized to the site of tumor.

- Diagnostic Approaches:
    - Clinical History: Progressive headache, associated neurological symptoms.
    - Neurological Exam: Thorough examination of cranial nerves, motor, sensory, reflexes, cerebellar, and cognitive functions.
    - Imaging: MRI of brain with and without contrast is the diagnostic study of choice.

- Pathophysiology: Mass effect, increased intracranial pressure, and local tissue damage.

11. Meningitis/Encephalitis

- Key Presentation:
    - Pain Characteristics: Severe, diffuse headache, often described as throbbing or constant.
    - Duration: Rapid onset of headache, typically within hours or days.
    - Associated Symptoms: Fever, neck stiffness, photophobia, altered mental status, seizures, rash in certain types of meningitis (e.g., meningococcal).
        - Meningitis: Inflammation of the meninges (membranes surrounding the brain and spinal cord).
        - Encephalitis: Inflammation of the brain tissue itself.
    - Pathophysiology: Infection of the meninges or brain tissue by bacteria, viruses, fungi, or parasites.
- Diagnostic Approaches:
    - Clinical History: Recent fever, headache, and change in mentation, any relevant travel history or exposures.
    - Neurological Exam: Assessment of mental status, meningeal signs (nuchal rigidity, Kernig's, Brudzinski's signs).
    - Lumbar Puncture: Analysis of cerebrospinal fluid (CSF) for cell count, glucose, protein, gram stain, and culture.
    - Imaging: CT head may be done prior to lumbar puncture to rule out increased intracranial pressure.

12. Idiopathic Intracranial Hypertension (IIH)

- Key Presentation:
- Pain Characteristics: Generalized headache, often worse in the morning, described as dull and pressure like. • Duration: Can vary from intermittent to constant. • Associated Symptoms: Visual disturbances (transient visual field changes, blurred vision,

diplopia), pulsatile tinnitus, papilledema, nausea. • Risk Factors: Obesity, especially in women of childbearing age.

- Diagnostic Approaches:
    - Clinical History: Headache characteristics, visual disturbances, tinnitus.
    - Neurological Exam: Assessment of visual fields, visual acuity, fundoscopic exam for papilledema, presence of any cranial nerve palsies.
    - Imaging: MRI or CT scan of the brain with and without contrast to rule out structural lesion, MR venography to see the venous system of the brain.
    - Lumbar Puncture: Elevated opening pressure on lumbar puncture.
- Pathophysiology: Increased intracranial pressure of unknown cause.

III. Comparative Summary Table

Feature	Migraine	Tension-Type Headache	Cluster Headache	Sinus Headache	Medication Overuse Headache	Cervicogenic Headache	Trigeminal Neuralgia	Giant Cell Arteritis	Subarachnoid Hemorrhage	Brain Tumor	Meningitis/ Encephalitis	Idiopathic Intracranial HTN
Pain Quality	Pulsating/ Throbbing, unilateral	Pressing/ Tightening, bilateral	Severe, sharp, unilateral, orbital/ temporal	Dull, pressure-like, bilateral	Variable, often continuous	Dull ache, unilateral, neck origin	Sharp, stabbing, electric shock-like, unilateral	Throbbing/ aching, new-onset	Sudden, severe, "thunderclap"	Progressive, variable	Severe, throbbing, diffuse, rapid onset	Dull, generalized, worse in AM
Pain Intensity	Moderate to severe	Mild to moderate	Severe	Mild to moderate	Mild to severe	Mild to moderate	Severe	Moderate to severe	Severe	Variable	Moderate to severe	Variable

Pain Duration	4-72 hours	30 min - 7 days	15-180 minutes	Days	Variable, continuous	Variable, can be constant	Seconds to minutes	Persistent, new onset	Variable, persistent	Increasing over time	Hours to days	Variable
Laterality	Unilateral (sometimes bilateral)	Bilateral	Unilateral	B lateral	Variable	Unilateral	Unilateral	Unilateral or bilateral	Diffuse	Variable depending on location	Diffuse	Bilateral
Associated Symptoms	Nausea, vomiting, photophobia, phonophobia, aura	Scalp/neck tenderness	Lacrimation, rhinorrhea, Horner's, restlessness	Nasal congestion, discharge, facial tenderness	Can have underlying headache features	Neck pain/ stiffness, limited ROM	Triggered by touch, chewing, can have sensory changes	Jaw claudication, visual loss, temporal tenderness	Neck stiffness, altered mental status, vomiting, focal deficits	Focal deficits, seizures, personality changes, papiledema	Fever, neck stiffness, altered mental status	Visual changes, pulsatile tinnitus, papilledema

Triggers	Stress, Diet, Hormonal, Sleep, Weather	Stress, muscle tension	Alcohol, odors, sleep disturbance	Upper respiratory infections, allergies	Frequent pain medication use	Neck movements, posture	Touching face, movements	Older age, history of PMR	Often spontaneous	Can depend on location	Infections	Obesity
Diagnostic Approach	Clinical history, ICHD-3 criteria	Clinical history, ICHD-3 criteria	Clinical history, ICHD-3 criteria	Clinical history, imaging if needed	Clinical history of medication use	Physical exam, cervical imaging	History, neuro exam, MRI scan	Clinical history, ESR/CRP, temporal artery biopsy	CT scan, clinical exam; possibly lumbar puncture	MRI Brain	Neurological exam, lumbar puncture	MRI, lumbar puncture

V. Key Takeaways

- Headaches are diverse: Understanding the numerous types of headaches is essential for proper diagnosis and treatment.
- History is crucial: A thorough patient history is the cornerstone of headache diagnosis.
- Red flags demand attention: Recognize life-threatening headache presentations, requiring immediate intervention.
- Differential diagnosis is paramount: Consider the various potential causes of headache symptoms.
- Diagnostic testing is targeted: Investigations are determined based on the clinical picture.
- Treatment is tailored: Individualized management plans are necessary for effective headache care.
- Underlying conditions must be considered: Headaches may be secondary to a more significant cause.
- Medication overuse can worsen headaches: Be mindful about analgesic use.
- Lifestyle plays a role: Stress management, regular sleep, and exercise can help prevent headaches.
- Recent research is advancing treatment: New options based on understanding of headache pathways are always emerging.

VI. Summary

The differential diagnosis of headaches is a complex endeavour, requiring a thorough understanding of various headache types, their clinical presentations, and appropriate diagnostic approaches. A systematic and personalized approach to headache management, incorporating a detailed history, comprehensive physical examination, targeted investigations, and tailored treatment strategies, will contribute to better patient outcomes. The ever-evolving landscape of headache research is bringing about new insights into pathophysiology and therapeutic interventions, which helps clinicians provide the most effective care.

VII. Bibliography (with Recent Research)

This bibliography includes recent research articles, guidelines, and textbooks to provide an up-to-date resource on headaches.

Journals

1. Cephalalgia: The official journal of the International Headache Society, publishes research on all aspects of headache.
2. Headache: The official journal of the American Headache Society, publishes peer-reviewed articles on all aspects of headache.
3. The Journal of Headache and Pain: Open-access journal covering headache research.
4. Neurology: Journal of the American Academy of Neurology, includes articles on neurological disorders including headaches.
5. JAMA (Journal of the American Medical Association): Publishes research articles, reviews on a wide range of medical topics including headaches.
6. Lancet Neurology: Publishes high-impact neurological research, including headache disorders.
7. PLOS ONE: Open-access journal publishing a broad range of science and medicine including headache research.
8. Annals of Neurology: Publishes original research in neurology.
9. Nature Reviews Neurology: Provides review articles and commentary on neurology topics.
10. Pain: Published by the International Association for the Study of Pain, covering chronic pain mechanisms and treatments.

Recent Research Articles

1. Edvinsson, L., Haanes, K. A., & Warfvinge, K. (2023). CGRP and migraine: From bench to bedside. Nature Reviews Neurology, 19(4), 221-234.
    - Overview of CGRP pathway in migraine, and the latest treatments.

2. Goadsby, P. J., & Deen, M. (2023). Cluster headache: recent advances and future directions. The Lancet Neurology, 22(10), 842-854.

    ○ Reviews recent advances in understanding the mechanisms and treatment of cluster headache.

3. Lipton, R. B., et al. (2022). Medication overuse headache: what have we learned and what do we still need to know? Cephalalgia, 42(8), 627-639.

    ○ Research on the pathophysiology, diagnosis, and mangement of medication overuse headache.

4. Ashina, M., et al. (2021). Cervicogenic Headache: A review of recent advances in diagnosis and clinical management. Cephalalgia, 41(7), 784-793.

    ○ Review of the diagnosis, pathophysiology, and management of cervicogenic headache.

5. May, A., & Schulte, L. H. (2021). The new classification of headache disorders The Lancet Neurology, 20(4), 233-234.

    ○ Commentary on the new edition of the International Classification of Headache Disorders.

6. Duh, L. et al. (2022). Redefining diagnostic criteria to improve detection of intracranial hypertension. JAMA Neurology, 79(12), 1215-1222.

    ○ An important paper that addresses the revised diagnostic criteria for IIH.

7. Afridi, SK., et al. (2022) Non-invasive vagus nerve stimulation in the treatment of refractory cluster headache using a hand-held stimulator. Cephalalgia, 42(14), 1322-133

Differential Diagnosis of Dizziness and Vertigo

Introduction

Dizziness and vertigo are common complaints that can significantly impact a patient's quality of life. These symptoms are not diseases in themselves but rather manifestations of an underlying pathology affecting the complex interplay of the vestibular system, central nervous system (CNS), and other sensory inputs. Accurately differentiating between the various causes of dizziness and vertigo is crucial for effective management, as the underlying etiologies range from benign and self-limiting conditions to serious and potentially life-threatening disorders.

This chapter provides a comprehensive guide to the differential diagnosis of dizziness and vertigo, focusing on key presentations, diagnostic approaches, and the distinctions among common etiologies. We will delve into the specifics of benign paroxysmal positional vertigo (BPPV), Meniere's disease, vestibular neuritis/labyrinthitis, migrainous vertigo, central causes of vertigo (including brainstem stroke, cerebellar ataxia, and multiple sclerosis), and acoustic neuroma. We will also provide a comparative summary table, key takeaways, a concise summary, and a bibliography with recent research to allow for a thorough understanding of this challenging area of clinical medicine.

Defining Dizziness and Vertigo

Before proceeding to the differential diagnosis, it is critical to define the key terms and their nuances:

- Dizziness: An umbrella term encompassing a range of subjective sensations, including light-headedness, faintness, unsteadiness, and disorientation. It can be further classified into:
    - Presyncope: The sensation of impending fainting, often due to decreased cerebral perfusion.

  - Disequilibrium: A sense of imbalance or unsteadiness, typically while walking.
  - Light headedness: A vague sensation of faintness, often described as feeling "out of it."

- Vertigo: A specific type of dizziness characterized by a false sensation of movement – either the individual is spinning (subjective vertigo) or the environment appears to be spinning (objective vertigo). It arises from an asymmetry in vestibular input. Vertigo is almost always indicative of a vestibular system disorder.

I. Benign Paroxysmal Positional Vertigo (BPPV)

A. Key Presentations:

BPPV is the most common cause of vertigo. It is characterized by:

1. Episodic Vertigo: Abrupt onset of intense vertigo attacks that are typically brief, lasting from seconds to a minute.
2. Positional Trigger: Vertigo is provoked by specific head movements or changes in head position, such as rolling over in bed, looking up, or bending down.
3. Nystagmus: Characteristic torsional and up beating nystagmus (in the posterior canal variant) or horizontal nystagmus (in the lateral canal variant).
4. Absence of Auditory Symptoms: Typically, there are no associated hearing loss, tinnitus, or ear fullness.
5. Latency: Usually, a brief delay of 1-40 seconds between the triggering movement and onset of vertigo and nystagmus
6. Fatigability: Repeated triggering manoeuvres will often result in a decrease or cessation of symptoms.

- Pathophysiology: BPPV is caused by the displacement of otoconia (calcium carbonate crystals) from the utricle into one of the semicircular canals, most commonly the posterior canal. The movement of these otoconia changes the endolymph flow and induces a false sensation of head movement.

B. Diagnostic Approaches:

1. Detailed History: An accurate history of symptom onset, duration, triggering factors, and associated symptoms is paramount.
2. Dix-Hallpike Test: The gold standard diagnostic test for posterior canal BPPV. It involves rapidly moving the patient from a sitting to a supine position with the head turned 45 degrees to one side and then observation of nystagmus.
3. Lateral Roll Test: Used to diagnose lateral canal BPPV. The patient is positioned supine, and the head is rapidly turned to one side, with observation of nystagmus.
4. Clinical Examination: Neurological exams should be unremarkable, excluding central causes.
5. Modified Epley manoeuvre: Can be utilized to treat BPPV by repositioning the otoconia back into the utricle

C. Differential Diagnosis:

- Central Positional Vertigo: This will have a persistence in nystagmus, not be direction-changing and not show latency or fatigability
- Orthostatic Hypotension: Presents with light headedness and presyncope rather than true vertigo.
- Other Peripheral Vestibular Disorders: Usually does not have episodic vertigo with changes in head position like in BPPV.

II. Meniere's Disease

A. Key Presentations:

Meniere's disease is an inner ear disorder characterized by:

1. Episodic Vertigo and Tinnitus: Attacks of vertigo lasting from 20 minutes to several hours (usually 2-3 hours) along with

fluctuating unilateral hearing loss, tinnitus, and aural fullness (a feeling of pressure or fullness in the ear).

2. Fluctuating Hearing Loss: Especially low-frequency, sensorineural hearing loss, which can progress over time.
3. Tinnitus: Low-pitched, roaring or buzzing tinnitus, often coinciding with vertigo attacks.
4. Aural Fullness: A feeling of pressure or fullness within the affected ear.
5. Vestibular symptoms such as nausea, vomiting, gait imbalance, and disequilibrium.
6. Interictal Symptoms: Some patients experience residual symptoms of dizziness or imbalance between attacks.

- Pathophysiology: Believed to result from endolymphatic hydrops, an excess of endolymphatic fluid within the inner ear, causing distention of the membranous labyrinth. The underlying cause of this is largely unknown.

B. Diagnostic Approaches:

1. Detailed History: Focus on the episodic nature of symptoms, associated auditory complaints, and duration of vertigo attacks.
2. Audiometry: Low-frequency sensorineural hearing loss is a characteristic finding.
3. Vestibular Function Tests: Caloric testing, video head impulse testing (vHIT), and vestibular evoked myogenic potential (VEMP) testing may show reduced function in the affected ear.
4. Electrocochleography (ECoG): Can sometimes demonstrate increased endolymphatic pressure.
5. Exclusion of Other Conditions: Ruling out other conditions such as acoustic neuroma, vestibular migraine, and autoimmune inner ear disease
6. MRI: Usually done to rule out other structural causes of these types of symptoms.

C. Differential Diagnosis:

- Vestibular Migraine: Can involve vertigo and tinnitus but is often associated with headaches and not hearing loss.
- Acoustic Neuroma: May cause unilateral hearing loss and tinnitus but typically doesn't present with episodic vertigo initially.
- Autoimmune Inner Ear Disease: Can cause progressive hearing loss and vertigo but usually does not have the specific episodic nature of Meniere's disease.
- Superior Semicircular Canal Dehiscence Syndrome (SSCD): Presents with sound induced vertigo and autophony

III. Vestibular Neuritis/Labyrinthitis

A. Key Presentations:

Vestibular neuritis and labyrinthitis are inflammatory conditions of the inner ear, distinguished by whether the inflammation only involves the vestibular nerve (neuritis) or also the cochlea (labyrinthitis).

1. Acute Onset of Vertigo: Sudden onset of severe, persistent vertigo that can last for days to weeks.
2. Nausea and Vomiting: Common symptoms associated with acute vertigo.
3. Postural Imbalance: Significant balance problems, making it difficult to walk or stand.
4. Nystagmus: Spontaneous, horizontal or torsional nystagmus, but typically beats away from the affected side.
5. Hearing Preservation (Vestibular Neuritis): Hearing is typically preserved in vestibular neuritis.
6. Hearing Loss and Tinnitus (Labyrinthitis): Labyrinthitis can involve hearing loss, tinnitus, and aural fullness.
7. No other neurological symptoms: The presence of neurological symptoms should always indicate a central cause of vertigo.

- Pathophysiology: Usually caused by viral infection (e.g., herpes simplex virus) of the vestibular nerve or the inner ear.

B. Diagnostic Approaches:

1. Detailed History: Sudden onset of sustained vertigo with associated symptoms.
2. Physical Examination: Nystagmus and postural instability with a negative Dix-Hallpike test and nystagmus that beats away from the affected side.
3. Head Impulse Test (HIT): Impairment of the vestibulo-ocular reflex (VOR) toward the affected side when performing a HIT while keeping the eyes fixed on a target.
4. Audiometry: Normal hearing in vestibular neuritis; sensorineural hearing loss in labyrinthitis.
5. Exclusion of Central Causes: A neurological examination is performed to rule out central causes of vertigo.
6. MRI: Usually done to rule out other structural causes of these types of symptoms.

C. Differential Diagnosis:

- Central Vestibular Disorders: More likely to have additional neurological symptoms, subtle nystagmus, and less severe vertigo.
- Meniere's Disease: Episodic nature of vertigo distinguishes it from the sustained vertigo of neuritis.
- Acoustic Neuroma: Typically has a more gradual onset and different pattern of hearing loss.

IV. Migrainous Vertigo (Vestibular Migraine)

A. Key Presentations:

Migrainous vertigo is a form of vestibular dysfunction associated with migraines. It is characterized by:

1. Episodic Vertigo: Vertigo attacks that may or may not be associated with headache, but should follow the pattern of a migraine (lasting 5 minutes to 72 hours).

2. Migraine Features: Often accompanied by other migraine symptoms, such as headache, photophobia, phonophobia, visual aura, and nausea.
3. Variable Presentations: The vertigo can be true rotational vertigo, light headedness, or a sense of unsteadiness.
4. Spontaneous or Triggered: May be spontaneous or triggered by common migraine triggers (stress, sleep deprivation, certain foods).
5. History of Migraines: A personal history of migraines and/or family history of migraines is usually present.
6. Symptoms between episodes Some patients report dizziness or brain fog in between episodes.
7. Duration of Vertigo: Episodes of vertigo can last from minutes to hours.

- Pathophysiology: The exact mechanism is unclear, but it is likely related to the interplay of neural pathways, neurotransmitters, and vascular changes in the brain during a migraine.

B. Diagnostic Approaches:

1. Detailed History: Focus on the association of vertigo with other migraine features, frequency of attacks, and presence of migraine triggers.
2. Diagnostic Criteria: The Bárány Society developed diagnostic criteria for vestibular migraine, which include vestibular symptoms coinciding with a history of migraines.
3. Neurological Examination: Neurological examination and testing are normal except in episodes.
4. Exclusion of Other Causes: Ruling out other vestibular disorders and neurological conditions.
5. Response to Migraine Therapies: Improvement with migraine-specific treatments can support the diagnosis.
6. Videonystagmography (VNG): Can identify both peripheral and central nystagmus.

C. Differential Diagnosis:

- Meniere's Disease: More clearly defined episodic nature with hearing loss, tinnitus, and aural fullness.
- BPPV: Vertigo is positional and not associated with migraine symptoms.
- Central Vestibular Disorders: More likely to have additional neurological symptoms.
- Vestibular Neuritis/Labyrinthitis: An acute, persistent nature of vertigo, not as episodic as in vestibular migraine.

V. Central Vertigo

A. Overview:

Central vertigo results from pathology in the CNS, including the brainstem and cerebellum. These conditions can be serious, requiring prompt identification and intervention.

B. Brainstem Stroke:

1. Key Presentations:
    - Sudden Onset Vertigo: Often severe and persistent.
    - Associated Neurological Deficits: Include diplopia (double vision), dysarthria (speech difficulty), dysphagia (difficulty swallowing), hemiparesis (weakness on one side of the body), ataxia (incoordination), and altered level of consciousness, which are key features distinct from peripheral vertigo.
    - Nystagmus: Direction-changing nystagmus that can be vertical, torsional, or horizontal, which is often not fatigable or suppressed with fixation.
2. Diagnostic Approach:
    - Neurological Examination: Thorough examination to identify focal deficits.

- MRI of the Brain: Imaging to confirm the stroke and identify the affected area.
- Vascular Evaluation: CT angiography or other vascular imaging to assess the blood vessels.

3. Differential Diagnosis: Other causes of stroke, including cardioembolic, or large vessel occlusive causes.

C. Cerebellar Ataxia:

1. Key Presentations:

   - Unsteady Gait: Characterized by a widened stance and irregular steps, difficulty walking in a straight line.
   - Ataxia: Incoordination of movements, particularly of the limbs, and difficulty with fine motor tasks.
   - Dysarthria: Slow, slurred, or irregular speech.
   - Nystagmus: Spontaneous nystagmus that can be horizontal, vertical, or rotatory that is not fatigable.
   - Vertigo: Often less intense than with peripheral disorders, more imbalance or disequilibrium.

2. Diagnostic Approach:

   - Neurological Examination: In-depth assessment of gait, balance, coordination, and speech.
   - MRI of the Brain: Neuroimaging to identify cerebellar pathology.
   - Underlying Etiology: Investigation into causes such as genetic disorders, autoimmune issues, toxins, or tumors.

3. Differential Diagnosis: Peripheral causes of vertigo, other causes of ataxia.

D. Multiple Sclerosis (MS):

1. Key Presentations:

    - Variable and Episodic Vertigo: Can present with vertigo, dizziness, or imbalance.
    - Other Neurological Symptoms: Fatigue, visual disturbances (optic neuritis), sensory changes, weakness, spasticity, and cognitive problems.
    - Relapsing and Remitting: Symptoms tend to occur in episodes or can be progressive.
    - Nystagmus: Often present as a central type nystagmus.

2. Diagnostic Approach:

    - Neurological Examination: Evidence of neurological deficits.
    - MRI of the Brain and Spinal Cord: Imaging showing demyelinating plaques.
    - Lumbar Puncture: Analysis of cerebrospinal fluid (CSF) for evidence of inflammatory markers
    - Evoked Potentials: Assessment of electrical activity in the brain and spinal cord to detect nerve damage
    - McDonald Diagnostic Criteria: Use of these criteria for diagnosis of MS.

3. Differential Diagnosis: Other causes of demyelination.

E. Pathophysiology:

Central vertigo is caused by disruption of the central vestibular pathways in the brainstem, cerebellum, or other areas of the brain.

F. Diagnostic Approaches:

1. Neurological Examination: A thorough neurological exam with particular attention to the presence of any other neurologic symptoms is critical.
2. Neuroimaging: MRI is the preferred method to visualize the brainstem, cerebellum, and other structures. CT scans can be useful in emergency situations.
3. Specific Tests: Additional tests may be indicated, based upon the suspected etiology.

G. Differential Diagnosis

1. Peripheral Vertigo: If nystagmus present, direction-changing and fatigable type nystagmus is diagnostic of peripheral vertigo.
2. Psychogenic Dizziness: Dizziness that does not fit any specific diagnosis.

VI. Acoustic Neuroma (Vestibular Schwannoma)

A. Key Presentations:

Acoustic neuromas are benign tumors of the vestibular nerve, specifically the Schwann cells.

1. Unilateral Hearing Loss: Progressive, often high-frequency, sensorineural hearing loss.
2. Tinnitus: Unilateral tinnitus in the effect ear.
3. Vertigo and Imbalance: Imbalance and/or disequilibrium is the more common symptom, with vertigo being less common and milder.
4. Cranial Nerve Symptoms: Larger tumors can cause facial numbness or weakness (trigeminal and facial nerve involvement).
5. Slow Progression: Symptoms usually develop slowly over time.

- Pathophysiology: Acoustic neuromas arise from the Schwann cells of the vestibular nerve, typically the superior branch and grow into the cerebellopontine angle.

B. Diagnostic Approaches:

1. Detailed History: History of progressive hearing loss, tinnitus, and dizziness symptoms are usually present.
2. Audiometry: Unilateral sensorineural hearing loss is a common finding.
3. MRI of the Brain with Gadolinium Contrast: Gold standard for visualizing acoustic neuromas and can show how much pressure it is putting on the surrounding structures.
4. Auditory Brainstem Response (ABR): Test to assess function of the auditory nerve and auditory pathways in the brain
5. Exclusion of Other Causes: Rule out other vestibular disorders.

C. Differential Diagnosis:

- Meniere's Disease: Episodic vertigo, fluctuating hearing loss, and aural fullness.
- Other CPA Lesions: Meningiomas and other masses in the cerebellopontine angle.
- Other Causes of Unilateral Hearing Loss: Sudden sensorineural hearing loss, autoimmune inner ear disease

Comparative Summary Table

Feature	**BPPV**	**Meniere's Disease**	**Vestibular Neuritis/Labyrinthitis**	**Migrainous Vertigo**	**Central Vertigo (Stroke)**	**Central Vertigo (Ataxia)**	**Central Vertigo (MS)**	**Acoustic Neuroma**
Vertigo Nature	Brief, positional	Episodic, lasts hours	Sustained, severe	Episodic, with or without headache	Sudden onset, severe	Chronic imbalance, less vertigo	Variable, episodic	Slow onset, chronic, often imbalance
Duration	Seconds to minutes	20 minutes to hours •	Days to weeks	Minutes to hours	Variable	Variable	Variable	Chronic
Trigger	Head movements	None, Spontaneous	Preceding viral illness	Migraine triggers	None, spontaneous	None, spontaneous	None, spontaneous	None, spontaneous
Associated Symptoms	None	Hearing loss, tinnitus, aural fullness	Nausea, vomiting, ± hearing loss (labyrinthitis)	Headache, photophobia, phonophobia, aura	Neurological deficits (diplopia, dysarthria, etc.)	Ataxia, dysarthria, incoordination	Fatigue, visual changes, weakness	Unilateral hearing loss, tinnitus, facial numbness
Hearing Loss	No	Fluctuating, low-frequency	Possible (labyrinthitis only)	No	No	No	No	Uniateral, progressive
Tinnitus	No	Present, low-pitched	Possible (labyrinthitis only)	Possible, but not prominent	No	No	No	Present, unilateral

Nystagmus	Positional, fatigable	Horizontal, may change direction	Spontaneous, horizontal or torsional	Variable, but usually horizontal	Direction-changing	Variable direction, not fatigable	Central type	Variable, direction changing
Dix-Hallpike Test	Positive	Negative	Negative	Negative	Negative	Negative	Negative	Negative
Head Impulse Test	No impairment	No impairment	Positive (if vestibular neuritis)	No impairment	No impairment	No impairment	No impairment	No impairment
Neurological Findings	None	None	None	None	Focal deficits	Ataxia, dysarthria	Various deficits	Late facial nerve involvement
Imaging	Usually not needed	Usually not needed	Usually not needed	Usually not needed	MRI: Often required	MRI: Required	MRI: Required	MRI: Required
Primary Cause	Otoconia in semicircular canals	Endolymphatic hydrops	Viral infection of vestibular nerve	Migraine-related mechanisms	Vascular event	Cerebellar pathology	Demyelinating plaques	Vestibular nerve tumor

Key Takeaways

1. Thorough History: The patient history is the most important aspect of the diagnostic approach to dizziness. Specific details of the symptoms, potential triggers, and timing of episodes provide essential clues.
2. Distinguish Vertigo from Dizziness: Accurately differentiate between true vertigo (rotational sensation) and other forms of dizziness (lightheadedness, presyncope, imbalance) as this guides the diagnostic process.
3. Peripheral vs. Central Vertigo: Identify whether the etiology is peripheral (inner ear) or central (brainstem, cerebellum) as central causes can be serious.
4. Nystagmus Analysis: The characteristics of nystagmus can be diagnostic or localizing.
5. Neurological Examination: A thorough neurological examination is critical for detecting central causes of vertigo.
6. Specific Diagnostic Tests: Utilize appropriate tests for each condition (e.g., Dix-Hallpike for BPPV, audiometry for Meniere's, MRI for acoustic neuroma).
7. Exclude Mimics: Be aware of conditions that can mimic vestibular disorders (syncope, orthostatic hypotension, anxiety, and other medical disorders).
8. Multidisciplinary Approach: Management of dizziness and vertigo may require collaboration with neurologists, otolaryngologists,

Bibliography:

- Textbooks:
  - Neurological Differential Diagnosis, by John Patten
  - Clinical Neuro-Ophthalmology, Fourth Edition, by Stephen J. Ryan and Jonathan B. Trobe

Differential Diagnosis of Seizures

Introduction

Seizures, characterized by transient alterations in brain function due to abnormal excessive synchronous neuronal activity, represent a common and concerning neurological event. While epilepsy, a condition marked by recurrent unprovoked seizures, is a primary consideration, many other conditions can manifest with seizure-like activity. Accurate and timely differential diagnosis is critical for appropriate treatment, management, and patient outcomes. This chapter will explore the key conditions that mimic seizures, focusing on their presentation, diagnostic approaches, and comparative distinctions.

Understanding Seizures: A Brief Overview

Before delving into differential diagnoses, it's important to briefly revisit what defines a seizure. Seizures are not diseases themselves but rather symptoms of underlying neurological dysfunction. They can range from subtle changes in awareness to dramatic convulsions. The International League Against Epilepsy (ILAE) classifies seizures into two primary categories:

- Focal Seizures: These originate within a specific area of the brain. These can be further categorized into:
    - Focal Seizures with Awareness (Simple Partial Seizures): Consciousness remains intact. Manifestations can include motor, sensory, autonomic, or psychological symptoms depending on the affected brain area.
    - Focal Seizures with Impaired Awareness (Complex Partial Seizures): Consciousness is impaired. Individuals may exhibit automatisms (e.g., lip-smacking, picking at clothes), and may be confused or unresponsive during the event.
    - Focal to Bilateral Tonic-Clonic Seizures: Begin as focal seizure that then spreads to include all of both hemispheres of the

brain, usually with loss of consciousness and tonic-clonic motor activity. Often referred to as secondarily generalized tonic-clonic seizures.

- Generalized Seizures: These arise from both hemispheres of the brain simultaneously. They include:
    - Tonic-Clonic Seizures (Grand Mal Seizures): Characterized by a loss of consciousness, followed by stiffening (tonic phase) and jerking (clonic phase) of both sides of the body.
    - Absence Seizures (Petit Mal Seizures): Brief episodes of staring and unresponsiveness without prominent motor activity. More common in children and adolescents.
    - Myoclonic Seizures: Sudden, brief jerks of muscles or muscle groups.
    - Atonic Seizures (Drop Attacks): Sudden loss of muscle tone, leading to falls.
    - Tonic Seizures: Sustained muscle stiffening without rhythmic jerking.

The etiology of seizures is broad, encompassing genetic, structural, metabolic, and immune factors. This chapter will focus on the entities that require differentiation from epilepsy.

Differential Diagnoses of Seizures

The primary conditions to differentiate from epilepsy include the following.

1. Epilepsy (Focal and Generalized)

Key Presentations:

- Recurrent, Unprovoked Seizures: The hallmark of epilepsy is a tendency for seizures to occur repeatedly without an identifiable, reversible cause. The International League Against Epilepsy (ILAE) defines epilepsy as at least two unprovoked seizures occurring more than 24 hours apart or one unprovoked seizure with a probability of further seizures similar to that following two unprovoked seizures occurring over at least 10 years.

- Varied Seizure Types: Epilepsy can manifest with any type of seizure described above. Understanding the seizure semiology (the characteristic features of a seizure) is extremely helpful in classification
- Aura: Some individuals may experience an aura—a warning sign experienced at the beginning of some focal seizures, such as a rising epigastric sensation, peculiar smells or tastes, déjà vu, or visual disturbances.
- Postictal State: Following a seizure, individuals often experience a postictal state characterized by confusion, fatigue, headache, or focal weakness (Todd's paralysis). The duration varies greatly depending on the type of seizure and the person.
- Interictal Period: Between seizures, individuals with epilepsy may have no symptoms or show subtle cognitive or behavioural changes.

Diagnostic Approaches:

- Detailed History: A thorough history, including a detailed account of the seizure event and associated signs and symptoms from the patient and witnesses, is critical. This aims to determine the nature of the seizure, any preceding aura, duration, and associated symptoms. Family history of seizures should also be noted.
- Physical Exam: A complete physical examination, including a detailed neurological exam, is critical to identify subtle findings indicating another disorder.
- Electroencephalography (EEG): EEG is a cornerstone of epilepsy diagnosis. It measures brain electrical activity. Interictal (between seizures) EEGs may show epileptiform discharges (spikes, sharp waves, spike-and-wave complexes) in those with epilepsy. Ictal

(during seizure) EEGs may capture the seizure activity which helps determine the type of seizure, its location of origin in the brain and may also allow for its differentiation from other causes. EEG may be limited by its ability to record only activity occurring on the surface of the brain, and its sensitivity is increased with longer durations of recording.

- Video-EEG Monitoring: Longer recordings of EEG paired with video can help capture and classify seizures, especially when they occur infrequently or are atypical.
- Neuroimaging: MRI of the brain is used to identify any structural causes of seizures, such as tumors, arteriovenous malformations (AVMs), cortical dysplasia, or hippocampal sclerosis. CT may be more readily available in the acute setting or if MRI is contraindicated, but is less sensitive than MRI for identifying subtle causes of seizures.
- Genetic Testing: In some cases, genetic testing may be indicated if there is a strong suspicion of genetic or familial epilepsy.
- Metabolic Testing: Labs should be obtained to evaluate for potentially treatable causes of seizures. These may include a complete metabolic panel, liver function, renal function, complete blood count, and appropriate toxicology screening.

2. Febrile Seizures

Key Presentations:

- Age-Specific Occurrence: Febrile seizures are nearly exclusive to children, primarily between 6 months and 5 years of age.
- Association with Fever: These seizures occur in conjunction with a fever greater than 38°C (100.4°F), not caused by a central nervous system infection.
- Generalized Seizures: Febrile seizures are typically generalized tonic-clonic seizures.
- Brief Duration: Most febrile seizures last less than 15 minutes.

- Simple vs. Complex:
  - Simple Febrile Seizures: Brief (less than 15 minutes), generalized, and occur only once within a 24-hour period.
  - Complex Febrile Seizures: Longer than 15 minutes, focal in nature, or occur more than once within a 24-hour period.
- Postictal Phase: Children may experience drowsiness or confusion after a febrile seizure.

Diagnostic Approaches:

- History: A detailed history of the illness, including the fever, associated symptoms, and characteristics of the seizure is important. The age of the child is crucial.
- Physical Exam: The examination focuses on finding the source of the fever, which may be a common infection like an upper respiratory infection, otitis media, or gastroenteritis. A neurological exam should be performed to rule out meningitis.
- Lumbar Puncture (LP): An LP is indicated if there is concern for meningitis, encephalitis, or if the source of fever is not apparent.
- EEG: EEG is generally not necessary for simple febrile seizures. It may be considered if there are complex febrile seizures or if there are concerns for underlying epilepsy.
- Neuroimaging: Neuroimaging is not routinely performed for simple febrile seizures, but may be considered with complex febrile seizures or if an underlying structural abnormality is suspected.

3. Psychogenic Non-Epileptic Seizures (PNES)

Key Presentations:

- Paroxysmal Events: PNES resemble seizures in that they involve sudden and temporarily altered behaviour and/or consciousness.
- Lack of Synchronous Neuronal Discharge: Unlike epileptic seizures, PNES are not caused by abnormal electrical activity in the brain.

- Variable Presentations: The clinical manifestations of PNES can vary widely, including motor activity (jerking, shaking), altered awareness, truncal movements (pelvic thrusting or head thrashing), apparent loss of consciousness, and vocalizations.
- Prolonged Duration: PNES can typically be longer in duration than epileptic seizures, often lasting more than 2 minutes.
- Dramatic Presentation: PNES may appear dramatic, particularly with forceful movements and crying, that may be disproportionate to the actual degree of physical distress.
- Lack of Postictal Confusion: A postictal period of confusion or fatigue is usually absent or significantly shortened compared to those of epileptic seizures.
- Eye Closure: During apparent loss of consciousness, patients with PNES often close their eyes tightly and resistant to opening.
- Pelvic Thrusting: Pelvic thrusting or head thrashing are common with non-epileptic seizures.
- Triggering Factors: PNES are often associated with psychological triggers, such as stress, trauma, or emotional distress.
- Coexisting Psychiatric Conditions: Many patients with PNES have comorbid psychiatric conditions, such as anxiety, depression, or PTSD.

Diagnostic Approaches:

- Detailed History: A thorough history from the patient and witnesses, including detailed descriptions of the events, potential triggers, and past medical or psychiatric history is important.
- Video-EEG Monitoring: Video-EEG monitoring is the gold standard for diagnosing PNES. It allows simultaneous observation of the clinical event and assessment of brain electrical activity. If the clinical event appears to be a seizure but there is no corresponding epileptiform activity on the EEG, PNES is the most likely diagnosis.
- Clinical Clues: The presence of certain clinical features increases the likelihood of PNES. These include asynchronicity

of motor activity, side-to-side head shaking, pelvic thrusting, weeping during the event, and closed eyes with resistance to opening.

- Psychiatric Evaluation: A psychiatric evaluation is important to identify any underlying psychological causes or comorbid conditions.

4. Syncope (Cardiac and Vasovagal)

Key Presentations:

- Transient Loss of Consciousness: Syncope is characterized by a transient loss of consciousness due to a temporary reduction in cerebral blood flow.
- Rapid Onset and Recovery: Syncope typically has a rapid onset and rapid recovery.
- Pre-syncopal Symptoms: Individuals may experience pre-syncopal symptoms such as light headedness, dizziness, diaphoresis (sweating), nausea, pallor, and visual changes (tunnel vision, greying out) before losing consciousness.
- Lack of Postictal Confusion: Although individuals can be disoriented just after syncope, they typically recover quickly to their baseline.
- Cardiac Syncope:
    - Sudden Collapse: Cardiac syncope may occur suddenly, with little or no warning.
    - Palpitations: Individuals may experience palpitations or chest pain before syncope.
    - Exertional Syncope: Syncope may occur during or after exertion.
    - Family History: A family history of sudden cardiac death is a potential risk factor for cardiac syncope.

- Vasovagal Syncope:
    - Provocative Factors: Vasovagal syncope is often triggered by emotional stress, pain, prolonged standing, or heat exposure.
    - Gradual Onset: Vasovagal syncope may have a gradual onset with preceding pre-syncopal symptoms.
    - Pallor: Patients may appear pale before losing consciousness.
    - Bradycardia and Hypotension: Vasovagal syncope is associated with a drop-in heart rate (bradycardia) and blood pressure (hypotension).

Diagnostic Approaches:

- Detailed History: Obtain detailed information regarding events leading up to and during the episode. Include details on activity during which the event occurred, time of day, positioning, and any triggering factors.
- Physical Exam: Assess vital signs, including blood pressure and heart rate. Auscultate the heart for murmurs and check for signs of hypovolemia.
- Electrocardiogram (ECG): An ECG is used to evaluate for cardiac dysrhythmias and structural cardiac abnormalities.
- Orthostatic Blood Pressure: Measurement of blood pressure and heart rate in both supine and upright positions.
- Tilt Table Testing: This test is used to assess for vasovagal syncope. During this test, the patient is placed on a tilt table and tilted to an upright position while blood pressure and heart rate are monitored.
- Echocardiogram: An echocardiogram may be indicated if cardiac pathology is suspected.
- Neurological Exam: To rule out any other neurological causes.

5. Hypoglycemia

Key Presentations:

- Neuroglycopenic Symptoms: Low blood glucose levels can cause a variety of neurological symptoms.
- Altered Mental Status: Hypoglycemia can cause confusion, disorientation, lethargy, irritability, and, in severe cases, loss of consciousness.
- Seizure-Like Activity: Hypoglycemia can manifest with convulsions or tonic-clonic activity that mimics seizures.
- Autonomic Symptoms: Hypoglycemia may cause autonomic symptoms such as sweating, tachycardia, palpitations, and tremors.
- Rapid Onset: The symptoms of hypoglycemia can develop rapidly especially if blood glucose drops abruptly.
- Improvement with Glucose: Symptoms should resolve quickly after blood glucose levels are corrected.

Diagnostic Approaches:

- Blood Glucose Measurement: A bedside blood glucose measurement should be performed immediately in any patient presenting with altered mental status or seizure-like activity.
- History: Obtain a history of diabetes, insulin use, or other risk factors for hypoglycemia.
- Physical Exam: Assess the patient for signs of autonomic dysfunction, such as diaphoresis.

6. Electrolyte Imbalances

Key Presentations:

- Varied Presentations: Electrolyte abnormalities can induce a range of neurological symptoms.
- Hyponatremia (Low Sodium): Hyponatremia can cause headaches, nausea, confusion, seizures, and, in severe cases, coma.

- Hypernatremia (High Sodium): Hypernatremia may cause irritability, confusion, seizures, and muscle twitching.
- Hypocalcemia (Low Calcium): Hypocalcemia can lead to muscle cramps, tetany, confusion, and seizures.
- Hypomagnesemia (Low Magnesium): Hypomagnesemia can cause muscle weakness, tremors, seizures, and cardiac arrhythmias.
- Gradual or Rapid Onset: The onset of symptoms may be gradual or rapid, depending on the severity and speed of the electrolyte change.

Diagnostic Approaches:

- Electrolyte Panel: Measure the levels of sodium, potassium, calcium, magnesium, and other electrolytes in the blood.
- History: Obtain a history of any underlying medical conditions, medications, or dietary factors that could contribute to electrolyte imbalances.
- Renal Function Tests: Assess renal function, which plays a crucial role in electrolyte homeostasis.

7. Drug Toxicity and Withdrawal

Key Presentations:

- Drug Toxicity: Overdose or toxic levels of certain medications can cause seizures including those medications with anticholinergic effects, local anaesthetics, and antidepressants. The specific symptoms will vary according to the specific substance.
- Drug Withdrawal: Sudden withdrawal from alcohol, benzodiazepines, and other sedative-hypnotics can cause seizures. Symptoms may include anxiety, tremors, agitation, and hallucinations.
- Timing Related to Exposure: Seizures may occur shortly after drug ingestion or during withdrawal from substances with sedative-hypnotic properties.

Diagnostic Approaches:

- Toxicology Screen: Perform a urine or blood toxicology screen to determine the presence of drugs or toxins.
- History: Obtain a thorough history of alcohol/drug use and medications that the patient is taking.
- Medication List: Review the patient's medication list to identify any potential medication-related causes of seizures.

8. Brain Tumor

Key Presentations:

- Focal Neurological Deficits: Brain tumors, particularly those in the cerebral hemispheres, often present with focal neurological deficits such as weakness, numbness, speech difficulties, or visual changes.
- Seizures: Seizures can be the first presenting symptoms of a brain tumor, particularly in the case of slow-growing tumors. The types of seizures may vary depending on the location of the tumor but can be focal or generalized.
- Headaches: Headaches, especially those that are new-onset, persistent, or worsening, may be a sign of a brain tumor.
- Increased Intracranial Pressure: Symptoms of increased intracranial pressure include headache, nausea, vomiting, papilledema (swelling of the optic disc), and altered mental status.
- Gradual Onset: Symptoms of a brain tumor typically develop gradually over weeks to months.
- Personality or Cognitive Changes: Brain tumors may cause changes in personality, cognitive function, or behaviour.

Diagnostic Approaches:

- Neurological Exam: Conduct a thorough neurological exam to identify focal deficits.

- Neuroimaging: MRI of the brain with and without contrast is the preferred imaging modality for diagnosing brain tumors. CT may be more readily available in the acute setting or if MRI is contraindicated.
- Biopsy: If a tumor is found, a biopsy will be necessary to determine the tumor type.

Comparative Summary

Feature	Epilepsy	Febrile Seizures	PNES	Syncope	Hypoglycemia	Electrolyte Imbalance	Drug Toxicity/ Withdrawal	Brain Tumor
Primary Cause	Abnormal neuronal activity	Fever	Psychological factors	Reduced cerebral blood flow	Low blood glucose	Abnormality in electrolytes	Exposure or withdrawal of substances	Structural lesion in the brain
Seizure Type	Focal or generalized	Generalized tonic-clonic	Variable (motor, apparent loss of consciousness)	Transient loss of consciousness with reduced muscle tone	Motor activity that resembles seizures	Variable (may be seizures)	Variable (may be seizures)	Can be focal or generalized
Consciousness	May be preserved or impaired	Usually impaired	May appear impaired	Loss of consciousness	Initially impaired, can lead to loss of consciousness	May be impaired	Varies	May be preserved or impaired
Duration	Variable	Usually <15 minutes, may be longer	Often >2 minutes	Usually <1 minute	Variable	Variable	Variable	Typically builds over time
Postictal Confusion	Common	Common but usually brief	Minimal or absent	Minimal or absent	Variable	Variable	Variable	Depends on the duration of the seizure activity

EEG	May have interictal epileptiform discharges	Typically normal after resolution	No epileptiform activity during events	Normal	Normal	May show non-specific abnormalities	May show non-specific abnormalities	May show focal slowing or epileptiform activity
Triggers	Unprovoked or provoked	Fever	Stress or emotional distress	Emotional distress, pain, prolonged standing	Inadequate glucose intake or medication imbalance	Underlying medical conditions or medications	Medications, drugs, or alcohol	Gradual onset, no specific trigger
Age	Any age	Usually 6 months to 5 years	Any age	Any age	Any age, especially in those with diabetes	All ages, particularly children and elderly	Any age	Any age
Other	Variable	Often associated with common infections	Often comorbid psychiatric conditions	May have pre-syncopal symptoms	Diaphoresis, tachycardia, palpitations	Muscle cramps or weakness	Anxiety, tremors, agitation	Headache, focal deficits, increased ICP

Key Takeaways

- Not all that looks like a seizure is epilepsy. It is essential to consider all other possibilities in the setting of acute changes in mental status with or without motor activity.
- A Detailed History Is Key: Taking a proper history from the patient and witnesses of the event will help the clinician make the appropriate diagnosis.
- Video-EEG Monitoring is Critical for PNES: This is the gold standard for diagnosing PNES and differentiating them from epileptic seizures.
- Cardiac syncope can be a cause of concern, particularly with those with history of sudden cardiac death in the family. ECG and cardiac testing are crucial.
- Promptly check blood sugar and electrolytes: These entities are potentially treatable and should be assessed for in anyone with concern for seizure activity.
- Consider substance use or withdrawal: Particularly in those with recent drug use or those with history of alcohol use.
- Neuroimaging should be done in those with suspicion for structural abnormalities: New onset seizures in adults need to have imaging performed to rule out a structural cause.

Summary

The differential diagnosis of seizures is a complex and essential aspect of clinical neurology. Conditions such as epilepsy, febrile seizures, PNES, syncope, hypoglycemia, electrolyte imbalances, substance use/ withdrawal, and brain tumors can all present with seizure-like events. A thorough history, detailed neurological examination, and appropriate diagnostic testing are necessary to establish the correct diagnosis and implement appropriate management strategies. It is critical to recognize the key differentiating features of each condition to ensure proper patient care and improved outcomes.

Bibliography

1. Gone Fisher, R. S., et al. (2017). Operational classification of seizure types by the International League Against Epilepsy: Position Paper of the ILAE Commission for Classification and Terminology. Epilepsia, 58(4), 522-530.
2. Scheffer, I. E., et al. (2017). ILAE classification of the epilepsies: Position paper of the ILAE Commission for Classification and Terminology. Epilepsia, 58(4), 512-521.
3. Berg, A. T., et al. (2010). Revised terminology and concepts for organization of seizures and epilepsies: Report of the ILAE Commission on Classification and Terminology, 2005-2009

Differential Diagnosis of Weakness

Introduction

Weakness, a ubiquitous symptom encountered across various medical specialties, often presents a diagnostic challenge. It can range from a subtle feeling of fatigue to profound paralysis, stemming from a myriad of underlying etiologies affecting the nervous system, muscles, or neuromuscular junction. This chapter aims to navigate the complex landscape of weakness, providing a detailed exploration of common causes, their key presentations, diagnostic approaches, and a comparative summary to aid clinicians in arriving at an accurate diagnosis and initiating appropriate management.

Understanding the Neuromuscular Pathway

Before delving into specific conditions, it's crucial to understand the neuromuscular pathway's basic components, whose dysfunction can manifest as weakness:

1. Upper Motor Neurons (UMN): These originate in the cerebral cortex and brainstem and project to the spinal cord, influencing lower motor neurons.

2. Lower Motor Neurons (LMN): Located in the anterior horn of the spinal cord and brainstem nuclei; they directly innervate muscles.
3. Peripheral Nerves: Transmit signals from LMNs to the muscles.
4. Neuromuscular Junction: The site where nerve terminals communicate with muscle fibers.
5. Muscles: The effectors that produce movement.

Dysfunction at any point along this pathway can result in weakness, with specific patterns and accompanying signs helping to narrow down the diagnostic possibilities.

Key Presentations of Weakness

Weakness can present in various patterns and characteristics, including:

- Acute vs. Chronic Onset: Sudden weakness (hours to days) suggests vascular events, inflammatory processes, or toxins, whereas gradual onset (weeks to months) may point toward degenerative, compressive, or chronic inflammatory conditions.
- Symmetrical vs. Asymmetrical: Symmetrical weakness typically involves systemic or diffuse processes, while asymmetrical weakness might indicate focal lesions.
- Proximal vs. Distal: Proximal weakness (difficulty raising arms or getting up from a chair) suggests myopathies, while distal weakness (trouble with fine motor skills or foot drop) may be due to neuropathies or neuromuscular junction disorders.
- Focal vs. Generalized: Focal weakness may be restricted to a specific limb or body part. Generalized weakness affects multiple muscle groups.
- Fluctuating vs. Constant: Fluctuating weakness that worsens with activity but improves with rest is characteristic of myasthenia gravis.
- Associated Symptoms: Accompanying symptoms such as sensory changes, pain, fatigue, muscle atrophy, autonomic dysfunction, or cognitive changes are crucial for differential diagnosis.

Differential Diagnoses of Weakness

Let's explore the common causes of weakness systematically, beginning with those affecting the central nervous system, then moving outwards:

1. Central Nervous System Causes: Stroke (Ischemic and Hemorrhagic)

- Key Presentation:
    - Sudden onset: Typically, within minutes to a few hours.
    - Focal neurological deficits: Weakness, numbness, or paralysis on one side of the body (hemiparesis/hemiplegia), facial droop, speech difficulties (dysarthria or aphasia), and vision problems.
    - Specific deficit patterns: Depend on the affected vascular territory of the brain.
    - Associated symptoms: Headache (especially in hemorrhagic stroke), altered consciousness, cognitive deficits.
- Ischemic Stroke: Caused by a blockage of a blood vessel in the brain, with common causes including thromboembolism from cardiac sources or atherosclerotic plaques.
- Hemorrhagic Stroke: Caused by a rupture of a blood vessel in the brain leading to bleeding within brain tissue or around the brain (subarachnoid hemorrhage).
- Diagnostic Approaches:
    - CT scan: Initial imaging of choice to differentiate between ischemic and hemorrhagic stroke.
    - MRI: More sensitive for detecting early ischemic changes and small lesions.
    - Angiography (CTA or MRA): To identify vascular occlusion or abnormalities
    - ECG and Cardiac Imaging: To evaluate potential cardiac sources of emboli.
    - Laboratory investigations: Including coagulation studies, lipid panel, glucose.

- Key Differentiating Features: Stroke is characterized by acute and focal deficits, in contrast to other conditions causing weakness. Hemorrhagic stroke typically presents with a sudden, severe headache, whereas this is less common in ischemic stroke.

2. Central Nervous System Causes: Transient Ischemic Attack (TIA)

- Key Presentation:
    - Sudden onset: Similar to stroke, but symptoms are transient, typically lasting a few minutes to an hour, and resolve completely within 24 hours.
    - Focal neurological deficits: Similar to those of stroke, including hemiparesis, dysarthria, aphasia, and visual disturbances.
- Pathophysiology: Temporary blockage of blood flow, typically due to a thromboembolism.
- Diagnostic Approaches:
    - Same as for stroke: CT/MRI, angiography, ECG, cardiac investigations, and laboratory blood tests.
    - Emphasis on identifying risk factors: Hypertension, diabetes, hyperlipidemia, smoking, atrial fibrillation.
- Key Differentiating Features: The transient nature of symptoms is the hallmark of TIA; however, it is regarded as a warning sign for future stroke.

3. Central Nervous System Causes: Multiple Sclerosis (MS)

- Key Presentation:
    - Variable presentation: Symptoms can vary widely depending on the area and extent of demyelination in the brain or spinal cord.
    - Relapsing-Remitting Pattern: Episodes of neurological deficits (including weakness, spasticity, fatigue, sensory changes, vision problems, bowel/bladder dysfunction) followed by

partial or complete recovery. May also present with primary progressive, or secondary progressive forms.
    - Optic neuritis: Can present as visual loss, pain on eye movement, and abnormal pupillary response.
    - Lhermitte sign: Electric shock-like sensations down the spine when bending the neck.
    - Uhthoff's Phenomenon: Worsening of symptoms with heat exposure.
    - Insidious onset: Symptoms develop over several days or weeks, often fluctuating in severity.

- Pathophysiology: Autoimmune-mediated destruction of myelin sheaths in the central nervous system, leading to disrupted neural signalling
- Diagnostic Approaches:
    - McDonald Criteria: Clinical presentation combined with evidence from MRI and cerebrospinal fluid (CSF) analysis.
    - MRI of the brain and spinal cord: Demonstrates characteristic white matter lesions.
    - CSF analysis: May show oligoclonal bands and elevated IgG index.
    - Evoked potentials: Assess the speed of nerve conduction.

- Key Differentiating Features: MS is characterized by relapsing and remitting symptoms, with brain and spinal cord lesions on MRI. Optic neuritis is a suggestive sign.

4. Peripheral Nervous System Causes: Guillain-Barré Syndrome (GBS)

- Key Presentation:
    - Ascending weakness: Starts in the legs and progresses to the arms, trunk, and facial muscles.
    - Symmetrical weakness: Affects both sides of the body equally.

- Areflexia/hyporeflexia: Loss or reduction of deep tendon reflexes.
- Sensory changes: Often present as tingling or numbness, but mild compared to the motor weakness.
- Autonomic dysfunction: Can cause fluctuations in heart rate, blood pressure, and bowel/bladder function.
- Rapid onset: Typically evolves over hours, days, or a few weeks.
- Preceding infection: Often history of respiratory or gastrointestinal infection prior to onset.

- Pathophysiology: Immune-mediated attack on the peripheral nerves, causing demyelination and axonal damage.
- Diagnostic Approaches:
  - Electromyography (EMG)/Nerve Conduction Studies (NCS): Demonstrate demyelination and slowed nerve conduction velocity.
  - CSF analysis: Increased protein with normal cell count (albumin cytologic dissociation).
  - Clinical history and physical examination: A key component in diagnosis.
- Key Differentiating Features: Rapidly ascending, symmetrical weakness with areflexia/hyporeflexia is highly suggestive. The absence of focal brain signs and the relatively prominent motor weakness, as compared to sensory symptoms, helps separate it from MS or stroke.

5. Neuromuscular Junction Causes: Myasthenia Gravis (MG)

- Key Presentation:
  - Fluctuating weakness: Worsened by activity and improved by rest.

  - Ocular weakness: Ptosis (drooping eyelids) and diplopia (double vision) are common early manifestations.
  - Proximal weakness: Affects upper and lower limbs more than distal muscles.
  - Bulbar weakness: Difficulty in speech (dysarthria), chewing, and swallowing (dysphagia).
  - No sensory changes: Pure motor presentation.
  - Fatigability: The weakness worsens throughout the day or during prolonged activity.

- Pathophysiology: Autoimmune-mediated attack on acetylcholine receptors at the neuromuscular junction, impairing muscle contraction.
- Diagnostic Approaches:

  - Acetylcholine receptor antibody test: Blood test showing positive antibodies in patients with MG.
  - EMG/NCS: Demonstrates decremental response to repetitive nerve stimulation.
  - Edrophonium(Tensilon)test:Ashort-actinganticholinesterase drug can temporarily improve weakness in MG.
  - Ice test: Improvement in ptosis after applying ice to the eyelid.

- Key Differentiating Features: Fluctuating weakness that worsens with activity and improves with rest, and often ocular symptoms, are characteristic. Repetitive nerve stimulation demonstrates decrement, helping to distinguish it from other conditions.

6. Peripheral Nervous System Causes: Neuropathy (Diabetic, Inflammatory, Compressive)

- Key Presentation:

  - Distal weakness: Usually affecting the hands, feet, or both.

- Sensory changes: Numbness, tingling, burning, or stabbing pain in the extremities (stocking-glove distribution).
- Muscle atrophy: In more chronic cases.
- Decreased or absent reflexes: Depending on the type and severity of neuropathy.
- Variable Presentation: The presentation of the neuropathy changes based on its underlying cause.

- Pathophysiology: Damage to peripheral nerves, caused by various factors such as metabolic disorders, inflammation, or compression.
- Types of Neuropathy and Diagnostic Approaches:
    - Diabetic Neuropathy: History of diabetes; often causes distal, symmetrical, and sensory-predominant neuropathy.
    - Inflammatory Neuropathies: (e.g., Chronic Inflammatory Demyelinating Polyneuropathy [CIDP]) Slower progressive cause of similar symptoms. EMG/NCS can demonstrate demyelination of peripheral nerves, with CSF showing elevated protein.
    - Compressive Neuropathies: (e.g., Carpal Tunnel Syndrome, Ulnar nerve compression) Focal symptoms of weakness in the specific distribution of nerve, with focal paraesthesia. EMG and NCS help confirm diagnosis.

- Key Differentiating Features: Distal weakness and sensory changes in a stocking-glove distribution are suggestive of peripheral neuropathy. The underlying cause, associated symptoms, and EMG/NCS findings help distinguish between different types. The presentation is generally more gradual than in conditions like GBS or stroke.

7. Muscle Causes: Myopathy (Muscular Dystrophies, Inflammatory Myopathies)

- Key Presentation:
  - Proximal weakness: Difficulty in climbing stairs, getting up from a chair, or raising arms above the head.
  - Symmetrical weakness: Muscles on both sides of the body are affected.
  - Muscle atrophy: May be present in chronic cases.
  - Fatigue & Muscle Cramps: Common symptoms in the myopathies.
  - No sensory changes: Pure motor involvement.
- Pathophysiology: Primary pathology of muscle tissue, due to genetic mutations, autoimmune reactions, or inflammatory processes.
- Types of Myopathy and Diagnostic Approaches:
  - Muscular Dystrophies: (e.g., Duchenne, Becker) Typically hereditary conditions with progressive muscle weakness. Elevated creatine kinase (CK), specific genetic testing can determine subtype.
  - Inflammatory Myopathies: (e.g., Polymyositis, Dermatomyositis) Autoimmune conditions with subacute onset. Elevated CK, positive autoimmune antibodies, muscle biopsy can be diagnostic.
- Key Differentiating Features: Proximal, symmetrical weakness and normal sensation point towards a myopathy. Elevated CK and underlying disease specific features help distinguish the specific subtype.

8. Motor Neuron Disease: Amyotrophic Lateral Sclerosis (ALS)

- Key Presentation:
    - Combined UMN and LMN signs: A mixture of weakness, spasticity, hyperreflexia, and muscle atrophy, fasciculations (muscle twitches).
    - Distal and proximal weakness: Often begins in one limb and can spread.
    - Bulbar involvement: Slurred speech, difficulty with swallowing, and tongue atrophy.
    - Progressive weakness: Symptoms gradually worsen over time.
    - No sensory changes or cognitive deficits: Initially, pure motor presentation.
- Pathophysiology: Degeneration of motor neurons in the brain, brainstem, and spinal cord.
- Diagnostic Approaches:
    - Clinical examination: To confirm motor signs consistent with ALS.
    - EMG and NCS: To detect denervation and fasciculations.
    - MRI of the brain and spinal cord: To rule out other causes.
    - Ruling out other mimics: Such as cervical spondylosis, myasthenia, myopathy.
- Key Differentiating Features: Combination of UMN and LMN signs, progressive weakness throughout the body (often starts focal) and the absence of sensory changes are important distinguishing features.

9. Spinal Cord Compression

- Key Presentation:
    - Variable symptoms: Depending on the level and extent of the compression.

  - Weakness: Can be localized to specific muscle groups innervated at or below the level of compression.
  - Sensory changes: Numbness, tingling, or paraesthesia below the level of compression.
  - Bowel and bladder dysfunction: Urinary retention, incontinence, or fecal incontinence.
  - Back pain: Can be a prominent symptom.
  - Spinal cord injury: Rapid onset of symptoms after trauma.
  - Tumor or epidural abscess: Slower onset of symptoms with potential systemic symptoms.

- Pathophysiology: Compression of the spinal cord or nerve roots due to trauma, tumors, abscesses, or degenerative conditions.
- Diagnostic Approaches:

  - MRI of the spine: To identify the location and cause of compression.
  - CT of the spine: Can provide initial information, especially in cases of suspected trauma or bony injury.
  - Myelography: When MRI is contraindicated.

- Key Differentiating Features: Symptoms often relate to a specific level of nerve compression and, in addition to motor deficits, tend to include sensory findings and bowel/bladder issues. Radicular pain with focal neurological findings is another suggestive symptom.

Comparative Summary of Weakness Etiologies

Feature	Stroke	TIA	MS	GBS	MG	Neuropathy	Myopathy	ALS	Spinal Cord Comp.
Onset	Sudden	Sudden	Insidious/ Relapsing	Rapid	Fluctuating	Gradual	Gradual	Progressive	Variable
Pattern	Focal	Focal	Variable	Ascending, Symmetrical	Proximal, Fluctuating	Distal, Symmetrical or Asymmetrical	Proximal	Mixed UMN/ LMN	Level-Specific
Weakness	Hemiparesis	Hemiparesis	Variable	Progressive; Areflexic	Fatigable; Proximal	Distal or Focal; Sensory-Predominant	Proximal	Diffuse	Specific Level
Sensory Symptoms	Variable	Variable	Common	Mild, Sensory changes	Absent	Common Sensory Changes	Absent	Absent	Present below Lesion
DTRs	Hyperreflexia/Absent	Normal/ Hyper	Variable	Decreased/ Absent	Normal	Decreased/ Absent	Normal	Hyperreflexia & Areflexia	Hyperreflexia/Absent
Other	Speech Deficits	Transient	Optic Neuritis	Autonomic Dysfunction	Ptosis, Diplopia	Pain, Tingling, Atrophy	Elevated CK	Bulbar Signs	Back Pain, Bowel/Bladder
MRI	Lesions	Negative	Lesions	Negative	Normal	Normal or can have enhancement	Normal	Can demonstrate atrophy	Cord Compression
EMG/NCS	Normal	Normal	Slowing	Demyelination	Decremental Response	Demyelination or Axonal Damage	Normal	Denervation, Fasciculation	Variable

Diagnostic Approaches: A Step-by-Step Guideline

The diagnostic approach to weakness should follow a logical sequence:

1. History:
    - Detailed description of weakness: onset, pattern, severity, associated symptoms.
    - Past medical history: Risk factors (HTN, DM, Smoking), prior CNS/PNS disorders, autoimmune conditions, family history of neurological diseases.
    - Medication history: including current medications and potential toxins.
    - Social and occupational history: to evaluate potential environmental or occupational exposures.
    - Any recent infection?
2. Physical Examination:
    - Complete neurological examination: Mental status, cranial nerves, motor strength, sensory function, reflexes, coordination, and gait.
    - General examination: looking for systemic signs (skin rashes, lymphadenopathy, weight loss).
    - Note pattern of weakness (proximal/distal, symmetrical/ asymmetrical).
    - Test for muscle atrophy, fasciculations, or myotonia.
3. Initial Investigations:
    - Blood work: Complete blood count, electrolytes, renal and liver function tests, glucose, inflammatory markers (ESR, CRP), thyroid function tests, vitamin levels (especially B12), and creatine kinase levels. Specific antibody tests (for myasthenia gravis, myositis, etc.) as clinically indicated.
    - ECG: To assess for cardiac arrhythmias or ischemia.

- Imaging:
  - CT of the brain: To rule out acute stroke.
  - MRI of the Brain/Spine: As appropriate to investigate the CNS more thoroughly.

4. Specialized Investigations:
   - EMG/NCS: To characterize and localize the site of nerve or muscle dysfunction (nerve vs. muscle vs. motor neuron disorders)
   - Lumbar puncture: CSF analysis for suspected infections, inflammatory, demyelinating conditions (GBS and MS)
   - Muscle biopsy: For suspected myopathies.
   - Genetic testing: For suspected muscular dystrophies or other hereditary conditions.
   - Tensilon test (Edrophonium): For suspected myasthenia gravis.

5. Reassessment and Follow-up:
   - Based on initial findings and response to treatment, a reassessment of the diagnostic plan.
   - Regular follow-ups to monitor disease progression, response to treatment, and need for further investigations.

Key Takeaways

- Weakness is a complex symptom: It can result from dysfunction at multiple levels of the neuromuscular system and requires thorough evaluation.
- Detailed History is Crucial: The onset, pattern, and associated symptoms are paramount to narrow the differential diagnosis.
- Neurologic exam: A thorough neurological exam with specific focus on identifying pattern of weakness, hyperreflexia vs hyporeflexia, muscle atrophy and sensory changes.

- Imaging: The use of imaging such as CT or MRI to rule out central nervous system causes is important in acute presentations.
- Specialized tests: EMG/NCS studies, Muscle biopsy, cerebrospinal fluid analysis help further distinguish between the differential diagnoses.
- Prompt and accurate diagnosis is crucial: Early identification allows for timely initiation of treatment and can improve outcomes.
- A systematic approach is key: combining clinical history, examination, and investigations in the correct order is the best way to arrive at an accurate diagnosis.
- Collaboration: working as a multidisciplinary team is essential for optimal patient care.

Summary

The differential diagnosis of weakness is a complex and demanding task, requiring a thorough understanding of the neuromuscular pathway and potential underlying conditions. This chapter has provided a comprehensive overview of common causes of weakness, their presentations, diagnostic approaches, and a comparative summary to aid in decision-making. By combining a detailed history, meticulous physical examination, and appropriate investigations, clinicians can navigate this diagnostic maze and provide effective management to patients experiencing weakness.

Bibliography (with Recent Research)

- Stroke:
  - Powers, WJ., Rabinstein, AA., et al. 2019 Guidelines for the Early Management of Patients with Acute Ischemic Stroke: 2019 Update to the 2018 Guidelines for the Early Management of Acute Ischemic Stroke. Stroke, 50(12), e344-e418.
  - Greenberg SM, Ziai W, Cordonnier C, et al. 2022 Guideline for the Management of Patients With Spontaneous Intracerebral Hemorrhage. Stroke. 2022;53(7): e282-e322. [(

Differential Diagnosis of Movement Disorders

Introduction

Movement, the seamless and intricate flow of our bodies, is a testament to the complex choreography of the nervous system. When this delicate orchestration is disrupted, a spectrum of movement disorders emerges, each characterized by distinct patterns of abnormal movements, posture, or tone. These disorders can profoundly impact an individual's quality of life, ranging from subtle tremors to debilitating involuntary movements. Accurate diagnosis is crucial for initiating appropriate management strategies, offering relief and potentially slowing disease progression. This chapter delves into the differential diagnosis of several common movement disorders, exploring key clinical presentations, diagnostic approaches, and distinguishing features to aid clinicians in navigating this challenging field. We will focus on Parkinson's disease, Essential tremor, Dystonia, Huntington's disease, Tardive dyskinesia, Restless legs syndrome, and Ataxia (both cerebellar and sensory), providing a comprehensive guide to their differentiation.

1. Parkinson's Disease (PD)

1.1 Key Presentations:

Parkinson's disease is a neurodegenerative disorder characterized by the progressive loss of dopamine-producing neurons in the substantia nigra, a region of the midbrain. This deficiency leads to a constellation of motor and non-motor symptoms.

- Motor Symptoms:
  - Resting Tremor: A hallmark of PD, this tremor is typically present when the limb is at rest, often with a "pill-rolling" appearance. It usually begins unilaterally and may eventually become bilateral.
  - Bradykinesia: Slowness of movement, which can manifest as difficulty initiating movement, reduced facial expression

(hypomimia), decreased arm swing when walking, and small, cramped handwriting (micrographic).
  - Rigidity: Increased muscle tone, often described as "cogwheel" rigidity when passively moving a limb. This rigidity affects both flexor and extensor muscles.
  - Postural Instability: Difficulty maintaining balance, often leading to falls. This symptom is usually a later manifestation of the disease.
  - Gait Disturbances: A shuffling gait with short steps and reduced arm swing, sometimes with festination (involuntary acceleration) or freezing (sudden inability to move).

- Non-Motor Symptoms:

  - Autonomic Dysfunction: These include constipation, orthostatic hypotension (low blood pressure upon standing), urinary urgency, and excessive sweating.
  - Cognitive Impairment: Problems with memory, attention, executive function, and mood disorders like depression and anxiety are common. Dementia can develop in later stages.
  - Sleep Disturbances: Insomnia, restless leg syndrome, and REM sleep behaviour disorder (acting out dreams) are frequently observed.
  - Sensory Changes: Reduced sense of smell (hyposmia or anosmia), pain, and paraesthesia can occur.
  - Fatigue: A pervasive and debilitating symptom.
  - Speech Problems: Hypophonia (soft speech), dysarthria (difficulty articulating words), and monotone speech.
  - Swallowing Difficulty: Dysphagia (difficulty swallowing) can occur, especially in later stages.

1.2 Diagnostic Approaches:

- Clinical Examination: A detailed neurological exam is the cornerstone of PD diagnosis. Observing the cardinal motor features, such as tremor, bradykinesia, rigidity, and postural instability, is essential.

- History: A thorough patient history of symptom onset, progression, and family history is crucial.
- Response to Levodopa: A significant improvement of motor symptoms after administration of levodopa (a precursor to dopamine) is a strong diagnostic indicator of PD. However, it's not a perfect test, as other parkinsonian syndromes can also show response.
- Imaging:
    - MRI: Usually normal in early PD but may help rule out other structural causes.
    - DaTscan: A single-photon emission computed tomography (SPECT) scan using an agent that binds to dopamine transporters is used to visualize the loss of dopamine terminals in the basal ganglia, supporting the diagnosis. It helps distinguish PD from Essential tremor or drug-induced parkinsonism which does not show such transporter loss.
- Blood Tests: There are no specific blood tests to diagnose PD, but these are used to rule out other conditions.
- Genetic Testing: Currently limited to specific cases where a genetic form of PD is suspected, such as early-onset PD or a strong family history.

2. Essential Tremor (ET)

2.1 Key Presentations:

Essential tremor is one of the most common movement disorders, characterized primarily by action tremor (tremor that occurs during voluntary movement). Unlike PD, the tremor is NOT worse at rest.

- Tremor:
    - Action Tremor: Present during voluntary movement, such as reaching for an object, holding a cup, or writing. It can be postural (when holding a position against gravity) or kinetic (during movement).
    - Bilateral: Usually affects both sides of the body, although can be asymmetric.
    - Frequency: Varies but usually fast (5-12 Hz).
    - Distribution: Primarily affects the hands and arms, but also common in the head (nodding or shaking), voice, and sometimes the legs.
    - Absence of Other Major Motor Signs: Unlike PD, ET does not exhibit bradykinesia, rigidity, or postural instability.
- Mild Course: ET is typically a slowly progressive disorder, and while it can be bothersome, it is rarely disabling.
- Symptom Worsening: Stress, fatigue, and caffeine or other stimulants can worsen the tremor. Alcohol can temporarily reduce the tremor in some individuals.
- Absence of Non-Motor Symptoms: ET does not typically involve cognitive impairment, autonomic dysfunction, or other non-motor issues like those seen in PD.
- Age of Onset: ET can occur at any age, but is most common in adults after age 40.

2.2 Diagnostic Approaches:

- Clinical Examination: Careful observation of the tremor during various activities is crucial, including testing for postural and kinetic tremor.
- History: Inquire about family history of tremor, as ET often has a genetic component. Pay attention to what medications the patient is taking, as some medications can cause tremor.

- Exclusion of Other Tremor Causes: Rule out conditions like Parkinson's disease, drug-induced tremor, hyperthyroidism, and cerebellar disease.
- Response to Medications: Beta-blockers (such as propranolol) and primidone are often effective in reducing tremor. These can serve as a diagnostic aid in the absence of conclusive tests.
- Imaging and Other Tests: Usually not necessary in typical cases. MRI is used if there is suspicion of a different cause for the tremor, and blood tests can determine if thyroid disease or other medical conditions are present.

3. Dystonia

3.1 Key Presentations:

Dystonia is a movement disorder characterized by sustained muscle contractions that cause repetitive twisting or distorting movements and abnormal postures.

- Involuntary Muscle Contractions: Sustained involuntary muscle spasms causing repetitive movements, twisting, or abnormal postures.
- Pattern of Movement: Can be focal (affecting one body part, such as blepharospasm - eyelid spasm, or torticollis which is neck spasm, or writer's cramp), segmental (affecting contiguous regions, such as the arm and neck), multifocal (affecting non-contiguous regions), hemi dystonia (affecting one side of the body), or generalized (affecting most areas of the body).
- Worsening with Voluntary Movement: Dystonia often worsens with attempted movement or specific actions.
- Overflow Phenomenon: Unintended muscle contractions in other body parts during intentional movement.
- Muscle Cramps: Can be painful and contribute to the atypical postures.

- Sensory Tricks (Geste Antagonist): Some patients find that specific tactile stimuli or manoeuvres can temporarily alleviate dystonia symptoms
- Variable Age of Onset: Can manifest in childhood, adolescence, or adulthood
- Fluctuations in Severity: Symptoms can vary throughout the day.
- Associated Features: Speech difficulties (dysarthria) and swallowing issues (dysphagia) can result from dystonic involvement of the muscles of the face, tongue, or pharynx.

3.2 Diagnostic Approaches:

- Clinical Examination: Observation of the characteristic posture and movements is the main diagnostic tool.
- History: A detailed history of symptom onset, progression, triggers, and family history should be obtained.
- Classification: Dystonia is classified based on its phenomenology, age of onset, and etiology (primary or secondary). Primary dystonia are often genetic; secondary dystonias typically have an identifiable underlying cause (e.g., drugs, stroke).
- Imaging: MRI of the brain may be done to rule out underlying structural lesions, especially in cases of secondary dystonia or atypical presentations.
- Genetic Testing: Useful in cases of primary dystonia, especially if there is a family history or early onset.
- Electromyography (EMG): Can confirm the presence of co-contraction of agonist and antagonist muscles, a hallmark of dystonia.
- Response to Treatment: Injecting botulinum toxin into affected muscles is one of the treatment options, and a positive response can also support the diagnosis.

4. Huntington's Disease (HD)

4.1 Key Presentations:

Huntington's disease is an autosomal dominant neurodegenerative disorder characterized by involuntary movements, cognitive decline, and psychiatric disturbances.

- Movement Disorder (Chorea):
  - Involuntary, jerky movements: Chorea is rapid, dance-like, and often unpredictable. It typically affects the face, limbs, and trunk.
  - Athetosis: Slow, writhing movements can also occur.
  - Difficulty with Motor Coordination: Problems with balance, gait, and fine motor skills.
  - Rigidity: Can develop in the later stages.
  - Bradykinesia: Slowness of movement can also occur
  - Dysarthria and Dysphagia: Speech and swallowing can be affected.
- Cognitive Decline:
  - Executive Dysfunction: Impaired planning, organization, and decision-making.
  - Memory Problems: Difficulty with short-term and long-term memory.
  - Slowed Processing Speed: Reduced ability to process information.
- Psychiatric Disturbances:
  - Depression: Very common.
  - Anxiety: Can be a significant problem.
  - Irritability and Aggression: May occur in some individuals.
  - Apathy: A lack of motivation or interest in activities
  - Obsessive-Compulsive Behaviours: Can be present.

- Family History: An essential feature, as the disorder is autosomal dominant, meaning that children of an affected person have a 50% chance of inheriting the disease.
- Age of Onset: Usually adult onset, typically between 30 and 50 years old. However, earlier or later onset can occur.
- Progressive Nature: HD is invariably progressive, leading to severe disability.

4.2 Diagnostic Approaches:

- Clinical Examination: Observation of the characteristic choreiform movements and assessment of cognitive and psychiatric symptoms.
- History: A careful family history is essential as it often confirms the presence of the disease in prior generations, since Huntington's is an autosomal dominant condition.
- Genetic Testing: The most definitive test is a DNA test to detect the genetic mutation (CAG repeat expansion) in the HTT gene.
- Imaging:
    - MRI: Shows progressive atrophy of the caudate nucleus and putamen, basal ganglia structures.
    - PET scan: May show reduced glucose metabolism in the basal ganglia.
- Cognitive Testing: Neuropsychological testing can assess the extent of cognitive impairment.
- Psychiatric Evaluation: To evaluate and manage the psychiatric symptoms.

5. Tardive Dyskinesia (TD)

5.1 Key Presentations:

Tardive dyskinesia is a movement disorder resulting from long-term use of dopamine receptor-blocking agents, such as antipsychotics and some antiemetics.

- Involuntary Movements:
  - Orofacial Movements: Typically involves the mouth, tongue, and jaw, causing facial grimacing, lip smacking, chewing motions, and tongue protrusion ("fly-catching" tongue).
  - Limb Movements: Choreiform (jerky) or athetoid (slow, writhing) movements of the limbs, sometimes including trunk involvement.
  - Stereotypical Movements: Repetitive and involuntary movements.
- Delayed Onset: Symptoms typically develop after months or years of exposure to dopamine receptor-blocking drugs.
- Variable Severity: Symptoms can range from mild to severe, with significant impact on daily life.
- Absence of Cognitive Impairment: Unlike Huntington's, TD usually does not involve cognitive decline.
- Potential for Irreversibility: While some cases are reversible after discontinuing the offending medication, TD may be persistent in many cases.
- Lack of Specific Treatment: Treatment options are limited and focus on managing symptoms.

5.2 Diagnostic Approaches:

- Clinical Examination: Careful observation of the characteristic movements.
- History: A crucial element is determining the patient's history of treatment with dopamine receptor-blocking drugs.
- Drug Withdrawal: Symptom resolution or improvement after drug withdrawal can support the diagnosis. However, this may not be feasible or desirable, depending on the medical situation.
- Differential Diagnosis: Ruling out other movement disorders, such as Huntington's disease, dystonia, or other drug-induced movement disorders.

- Standardized Rating Scales: Scales like the Abnormal Involuntary Movement Scale (AIMS) are used to monitor the severity of TD.
- Imaging: Usually not helpful in TD unless ruling out other causes is needed.

6. Restless Legs Syndrome (RLS)

6.1 Key Presentations:

Restless legs syndrome (RLS) is characterized by an urge to move the legs due to unpleasant sensations, often described as crawling, tingling, or pulling sensations.

- Urge to Move Legs: An irresistible urge to move the legs, often accompanied by uncomfortable sensations.
- Symptoms Worsening at Rest: Symptoms are typically worse during periods of inactivity or rest, especially in the evening or at night.
- Temporary Relief with Movement: Symptoms are usually relieved by movement, such as walking or stretching.
- Circadian Pattern: Symptoms are often more prominent in the evening or at night.
- Periodic Limb Movements in Sleep (PLMS): Involuntary leg jerks during sleep, often disrupting sleep quality.
- Sleep Disturbance: Insomnia and daytime sleepiness can result from poor sleep quality.
- Primary or Secondary: RLS can be primary (idiopathic) or secondary to other conditions (e.g., iron deficiency, pregnancy, kidney failure, peripheral neuropathy).
- Family History: It often runs in families.

6.2 Diagnostic Approaches:

- Clinical Diagnosis: Diagnosis is primarily clinical, based on the patient's description of symptoms. The International Restless Legs Syndrome (IRLS) study group diagnostic criteria, require the presence of all 5 essential criteria:

1. An urge to move the legs, usually associated with unpleasant sensations
2. The urge to move begins or worsens during periods of rest or inactivity.
3. The urge is partially or totally relieved by movement
4. The urge to move occurs during evening or at night rather than during the day.
5. These symptoms are not due to another medical or behavioural disorder.

- History: A detailed history of symptoms, family history, medications, and other medical conditions is essential.
- Iron Studies: Ferritin levels should be checked to identify iron deficiency, a common cause of secondary RLS.
- Sleep Studies (Polysomnography): May be done to confirm PLMS and evaluate sleep quality, particularly if a specific sleep disorder is suspected.
- Electrodiagnostic Studies: Rarely needed. Nerve conduction studies can be done in cases where neuropathy is suspected.
- Differential Diagnosis: Ruling out other conditions causing similar symptoms, such as neuropathy, vascular issues, radiculopathy, or positional discomfort.
- Response to Treatment: A therapeutic trial with medications for RLS can be an adjunct to diagnostics.

7. Ataxia (Cerebellar and Sensory)

7.1 Key Presentations:

Ataxia is a movement disorder characterized by a lack of coordination and balance, resulting from dysfunction of the cerebellum or sensory pathways. Distinguishing between cerebellar and sensory ataxia is crucial.

7.1.1 Cerebellar Ataxia:

- Gait Ataxia: Wide-based gait with unsteady, staggering movements.
- Limb Ataxia: Poor coordination and dysmetria (inaccuracy in reaching movements) when reaching for objects or performing skilled movements.
- Intention Tremor: Tremor that worsens as the limb approaches a target.
- Dysdiadochokinesia: Difficulty performing rapid alternating movements (e.g., pronation and supination of the forearms).
- Dysarthria: Slurred, scanned speech.
- Nystagmus: Involuntary eye movements.
- Hypotonia: Reduced muscle tone may be present
- Balance Problems: Difficulty maintaining balance, especially during gait or standing.

7.1.2 Sensory Ataxia:

- Loss of Proprioception: Difficulty knowing the position of the limbs in space, leading to uncoordinated, clumsy movements.
- Gait Ataxia: Unsteady, high-stepping gait, often with stomping movements.
- Romberg Sign: Loss of balance when standing with feet together and eyes closed.
- Pseudo athetosis: Involuntary writhing movements of the fingers and hands, particularly when the eyes are closed.
- Loss of Vibration Sense: Reduced ability to perceive vibration in the extremities.
- Absence of Cerebellar Signs: No nystagmus, intention tremor, or dysdiadochokinesia.

7.2 Diagnostic Approaches:

- Clinical Examination: Detailed neurological examination, focusing on gait, limb coordination, balance, and sensory function.

- History: Details about the onset, progression, and associated symptoms, including any family history of ataxia.
- Imaging:
    - MRI of the Brain and Spinal Cord to evaluate for structural lesions, cerebellar atrophy, or spinal cord disease.
    - CT scan may be used if MRI is contra-indicated or not available.
- Electrophysiology: Nerve conduction studies and EMG can identify peripheral neuropathy, which may contribute to sensory ataxia.
- Blood Tests: To identify underlying causes such as vitamin deficiencies (B12, E), hypothyroidism, celiac disease, or genetic conditions.
- Genetic Testing Specific genetic tests for various hereditary ataxias, if indicated by family history or clinical presentation.
- Cerebrospinal Fluid Analysis To rule out inflammatory causes and infectious causes.

8. Comparative Summary

To highlight the distinctions between these movement disorders, a comparative summary table is presented below:

Feature	Parkinson's Disease	Essential Tremor	Dystonia	Huntington's Disease	Tardive Dyskinesia	Restless Legs Syndrome	Cerebellar Ataxia	Sensory Ataxia
Primary Tremor	Resting, "pill-rolling"	Action (postural/kinetic)	Not a primary feature	Not a primary feature	Not usually a tremor but facial / limb movements	Not a primary feature	Intention tremor, rarely present at rest	No tremor
Bradykinesia	Present	Absent	Absent, slowness secondary to abnormal posture.	Present	Absent	Absent	May occur but less characteristic	Absent
Rigidity	Present	Absent	Present	Present	Absent	Absent	May occur but less characteristic	Absent
Postural Instability	Present	Absent	Not consistent with Dystonia	Present	Absent	Absent	Present	Variable
Involuntary Movements	Absent (except tremor)	Absent	Twisting, abnormal posture	Chorea, athetosis	Orofacial, limb, and truncal	Urge to move legs	Uncoordinated movements	Clumsy, uncoordinated movements
Cognitive Impairment	Common, especially late	Absent	Absent	Present, often progressive	Absent	Absent	May occur	Secondary to Sensory Loss
Onset	Usually late adult	Any age but usually older adults	Variable	Adult onset, usually after 30-50 years	Delayed onset after long term use of offending agent	Often in adults	Variable, depending on the cause	Variable, depending on the cause

Family History	Sometimes	Often	Sometimes	Usually Present (autosomal dominant)	Usually Absent	Often Present	Present in hereditary forms	Cause-dependent, can be present in some conditions
Response to Levodopa	Usually good	None	Variable	None	None	Variable	None	Variable
Association	Dopamine Deficiency/ Loss of Substantia Nigra	Genetic factors	Genetic/Environmental/ Drug-induced, basal ganglia dysfunction	Genetic- CAG repeats in gene	Prolonged use of dopamine receptor blockers	Iron deficiency, genetic components	Cerebellar injury, genetic components	Loss of proprioceptive input from sensory nerves, spinal cord, or brain.

9. Key Takeaways

- Clinical Presentation is Key: Careful observation of movement patterns, timing, and associated features is paramount for differential diagnosis.
- History, History, History: A thorough patient history is essential, focusing on symptom onset, progression, family history, drug use, and co-morbidities.
- Consider Multiple Disorders: Patients may present with features overlapping different movement disorders, necessitating meticulous assessment.
- Rule Out Treatable Causes: Always consider secondary causes (e.g., medication-

Bibliography

1. Jankovic, J. (2008). Parkinson's disease: clinical features and diagnosis. Journal of neurology, neurosurgery, and psychiatry, 79(4), 368-376.
2. Bhatia, K. P., & Bain, P. (2014). A review of essential tremor. Journal of Neurology, Neurosurgery & Psychiatry, 85(11), 1287-1293.
3. Albanese, A., Bhatia, K. P., & Bressman, S. B. (2012). Phenomenology and classification of dystonia: a consensus update. Movement Disorders, 27(7), 863-873.
4. McColgan, P., & Tabrizi, S. J. (2018). Huntington's disease: a clinical review. European journal of neurology, 25(1), 24-34.
5. Kulkarni, R., & Jeste, D. V. (2022). Tardive dyskinesia: prevalence, clinical features, risk factors, and management strategies. CNS drugs, 36(8), 801-820.
6. Allen, R. P., Picchietti, D. L., Garcia-Borre Guero, D., Ondo, W. G., Walter, A. S., Winkelman, J. W., & Trenk Walder, C. (2014). Restless legs syndrome/Willis-Ekbom disease diagnostic criteria: updated International Restless Legs Syndrome Study Group

(IRLSSG) consensus criteria–history, rationale, description, and significance. Sleep Medicine, 15(6), 615-625.
7. Hoche, F., & Timmann, D. (2022). Cerebellar ataxia. Handbook of Clinical Neurology, 187, 45-60.
8. Manto, M., & Grunewald, R. (2013). Sensory ataxia. Handbook of Clinical Neurology, 116, 289-302.

Differential Diagnosis of Visual Disturbances

Introduction

The visual system, a marvel of biological engineering, relies on a complex interplay of structures, from the cornea and lens to the retina, optic nerve, and visual cortex. Disturbances at any point along this pathway can manifest as a wide array of visual symptoms, ranging from subtle blurring to complete loss of sight. A systematic approach to differential diagnosis is crucial for accurately identifying the underlying pathology and guiding appropriate management. This chapter provides an in-depth exploration of several common and clinically significant visual disturbances, covering their key presentations, diagnostic approaches, a comparative summary, and important takeaways for clinicians.

1. Optic Neuritis: Inflammation of the Visual Pathway

Optic neuritis (ON) is an inflammatory demyelinating condition affecting the optic nerve, the pathway that transmits visual information from the eye to the brain. It is a common cause of acute vision loss, particularly in younger adults.

- Key Presentations:
    - Acute Vision Loss: Typically develops rapidly over hours to days, often in one eye.
    - Pain: Retro-orbital pain, often exacerbated by eye movements, is a characteristic feature.
    - Dyschromatopsia: Decreased color vision, particularly red-green discrimination.

- Afferent Pupillary Defect (APD): A relative afferent pupillary defect is present in unilateral cases. The affected pupil does not constrict well when light is shone into it compared to the unaffected eye.
- Visual Field Defects: A variety of defects may occur, such as a central scotoma (blind spot in the centre of vision), but any pattern is possible.
- Uhthoff Phenomenon: Transient worsening of vision with increases in body temperature (e.g., after exercise or hot bath).

- Diagnostic Approaches:
  - Ophthalmoscopy: May reveal optic disc swelling (papillitis) in about one-third of cases, particularly in the acute phase. The optic disc may appear normal in retrobulbar neuritis.
  - Visual Field Testing: Formal testing to document the specific patterns of visual field loss.
  - Optical Coherence Tomography (OCT): Can quantify retinal nerve fibre layer (RNFL) swelling and thinning. In acute phase will be increased and then after a few months will thin.
  - Magnetic Resonance Imaging (MRI) of the Brain and Orbits: Crucial to identify the presence of demyelinating lesions in the optic nerve. T2 weighted sequences will show hyperintensity of the optic nerve. MRI is also critical for evaluating for underlying multiple sclerosis (MS) where brain lesions may be present.
  - Visual Evoked Potentials (VEP): Demonstrates delayed conduction along the optic nerve.
  - Lumbar Puncture: May be indicated to assess for oligoclonal bands in CSF in suspected MS.
  - Blood Tests: May be indicated to look for causes like neuromyelitis Optica, systemic inflammatory or infectious diseases

- Differential Diagnoses:
  - Papilledema: Disc swelling due to raised intracranial pressure. Optic neuritis will often present with pain and vision loss, both of which are typically absent in papilledema
  - Anterior Ischemic Optic Neuropathy (AION): Usually in older adults, without pain and more sudden onset and does not typically improve over time.
  - Compressive Optic Neuropathy: Caused by tumors or other masses impinging on the optic nerve. Typically has a more protracted course and gradual onset vision loss
  - Leber Hereditary Optic Neuropathy (LHON): Inherited disorder causing bilateral vision loss.
  - Infectious Optic Neuritis: Caused by infections such as tuberculosis, Lyme disease, syphilis and others.
  - Sarcoidosis: Granulomatous inflammation of the optic nerve
- Treatment & Key Takeaways:
  - The primary goal of treatment is to decrease inflammation and the duration of acute vision loss.
  - Intravenous high dose corticosteroids may be considered.
  - Early diagnosis and prompt initiation of treatment can result in faster visual recovery
  - Patients with optic neuritis will have a higher risk of developing multiple sclerosis in the future

2. Papilledema: The Swollen Optic Disc

Papilledema refers to optic disc swelling secondary to increased intracranial pressure (ICP), which can be caused by various conditions affecting the brain and its surroundings.

- Key Presentations:
  - Bilateral Optic Disc Swelling: Usually involves both eyes, but asymmetry can occur.

- Enlarged Blind Spot: Commonly present due to the optic disc edema.
- Transient Visual Obscuration: Brief episodes of vision loss, often lasting just a few seconds and may be provoked by changes in position.
- Headache: May be present, often worse in the morning, or with Valsalva manoeuvres.
- Nausea/Vomiting: May accompany headache due to raised intracranial pressure.
- Pulsatile Tinnitus: A whooshing sound in the ears may be present.

- Diagnostic Approaches:
  - Ophthalmoscopy: Classic finding of bilateral disc swelling.
    - Blurring of the disc margins, often with peripapillary hemorrhage.
    - Elevation of the optic disc, resulting in a "champagne cork" appearance.
    - Venous engorgement and tortuosity of retinal vessels.
  - Visual Field Testing: For early or subtle cases, this can show an enlargement of the blind spot.
  - MRI of the Brain: Imaging is critical to rule out intracranial masses, hydrocephalus, and cerebral venous thrombosis.
  - Lumbar Puncture: To measure the cerebrospinal fluid (CSF) pressure and analyse the CSF for signs of infection or inflammation.
  - Optical Coherence Tomography (OCT): OCT Can determine the level of retinal nerve fibre layer swelling.
- Differential Diagnoses:
  - Optic Neuritis: Distinguished by pain on eye movements, afferent pupillary defect, and usually unilateral.

    - Pseudo-papilledema: Apparent disc swelling secondary to optic disc drusen or other anatomical variations. Usually there is not true disc edema as assessed via OCT.
    - Ischemic Optic Neuropathy: Typically, presents with sudden unilateral vision loss without headache.
    - Malignant hypertension: Associated with severe hypertension.
    - Other causes of optic disc swelling: Such as infiltrative/ inflammatory processes

- Key Takeaways:
    - Papilledema is a sign of increased ICP which is secondary to an underlying condition
    - Prompt diagnosis and treatment of the underlying cause is essential to prevent irreversible visual loss.
    - Lumbar puncture is critical to document increased ICP.
    - Imaging should be obtained urgently to rule out mass lesions.
    - Management is dependent on underlying etiology such as removal of mass lesion or medications to decrease ICP.

3. Visual Field Defects: Mapping the Blind Spots

Visual field defects are limitations in the normal field of vision caused by lesions anywhere along the visual pathway, from the retina to the occipital lobe. They can present with various patterns, offering valuable clues about the location of the underlying pathology. Hemianopia and quadrantanopia are two of the most clinically relevant patterns.

- Hemianopia:
    - Definition: Loss of vision in one half of the visual field.
    - Types:
        - Homonymous Hemianopia: Loss of vision in the same side of the visual field in both eyes (e.g., loss of the right

visual field in both eyes). Typically seen with lesions in the retro chiasmatic pathway.

- Heteronymous Hemianopia: Loss of vision in different halves of the visual field in each eye.
    - Bitemporal Hemianopia: Loss of vision in the outer (temporal) half of the visual field in each eye. Most common cause is chiasmal lesions like pituitary tumors
    - Binassal Hemianopia: Loss of vision in the inner (nasal) half of the visual field in each eye. This is rare and is usually caused by lesions that compress on both sides of the optic chiasm.

- Key Presentations:
    - Patient may report bumping into objects on one side or difficulty judging spatial relations.
    - May be unaware of the deficit, especially if it's slowly progressive.

- Quadrantanopia:
    - Definition: Loss of vision in one quadrant of the visual field.
    - Types:
        - Homonymous Superior Quadrantanopia: Loss of vision in the upper quadrant on the same side of the visual field in both eyes. Usually related to lesions of optic radiations in temporal lobe
        - Homonymous Inferior Quadrantanopia: Loss of vision in the lower quadrant on the same side of the visual field in both eyes. Usually related to lesions of optic radiations in parietal lobe

- Key Presentations:
  - Similar to hemianopia, but visual field deficit involves only a quarter of the visual field.

- Diagnostic Approaches:
  - Confrontation Visual Field Testing: A quick method to test for large field defects
  - Automated Perimetry: Quantitative, objective assessment of visual field using specific targets. This is the most common method for formalized visual field testing.
  - Ophthalmologic Examination: Evaluation of the retina and optic nerve for local causes of field loss
  - Neuroimaging (MRI or CT): To identify underlying central nervous system pathology.

- Differential Diagnoses:
  - Glaucoma: Can cause peripheral field loss, typically not respecting the vertical midline.
  - Retinal Conditions: Such as retinitis pigmentosa, retinal detachment and retinal artery occlusion
  - Optic Neuropathies: Lesions of optic nerve can cause a variety of defects, often including central scotoma
  - Stroke/Vascular Events: Common cause of homonymous defects.
  - Tumors: Can compress on any part of the visual pathway.
  - Multiple Sclerosis: Can cause field defects due to demyelinating lesions.

- Key Takeaways:
  - The exact type of visual field defect points to the location of the lesion along the visual pathway e.g. lesions of the lateral geniculate nucleus will result in incongruous homonymous

hemianopia and lesions of the optic radiations will result in a congruous homonymous hemianopia

- Homonymous defects are always caused by retro chiasmal lesions
- Bitemporal Hemianopia is most commonly secondary to chiasmal lesions.
- Accurate visual field testing and neuroimaging are critical for diagnosis.
- Management depends on the underlying cause.

4. Double Vision (Diplopia): A Disturbance of Binocular Vision

Diplopia, or double vision, occurs when the visual axes of the two eyes are not aligned, resulting in the perception of two images of a single object.

- Key Presentations:
  - Monocular Diplopia: Double vision presents in one eye. Typically, due to refractive errors, dry eye syndrome, or cataract.
  - Binocular Diplopia: Double vision presents when both eyes are open, but resolves when either eye is covered. Due to misalignment of the eyes.
    - Horizontal Diplopia: Double images are side by side. Indicative of medial or lateral rectus muscle impairment.
    - Vertical Diplopia: Double images are one above the other. Indicative of superior or inferior rectus/oblique muscle impairment.
    - Oblique Diplopia: Double images are diagonal.
- Diagnostic Approaches:
  - Detailed History: Onset, duration, associated symptoms, alleviating factors.

- Ophthalmic Examination:
  - Assessment of pupil size and reactivity.
  - Check for ptosis (drooping eyelid) which may be associated with a third nerve palsy.
  - Motility testing to document the extent of extraocular muscle movement in each eye.
  - Cover test to quantify deviation (strabismus).
- Neurological Examination: To look for any other signs of underlying neurological deficits.
- Neuroimaging (MRI or CT): May be required if neurological cause is identified.
- Blood tests: May be indicated to look for thyroid disease, myasthenia gravis, or other inflammatory conditions.

- Differential Diagnoses:
  - Third Nerve Palsy: Affects eye movements, pupillary constriction, and eyelid elevation. Ptosis is often present.
  - Fourth Nerve Palsy: Affects vertical and torsional eye movements, causing vertical diplopia. Patient may complain of head tilt.
  - Sixth Nerve Palsy: Affects ability to abduct (move eye outward) and causes horizontal diplopia.
  - Myasthenia Gravis: Autoimmune condition causing muscle weakness, including the extraocular muscles. Symptoms worsen with fatigue.
  - Thyroid Eye Disease: Autoimmune disease that results in swelling of muscles surrounding the eye.
  - Orbital Mass or Inflammation: Can impinge on the extraocular muscles.
  - Intracranial lesions: Brainstem strokes, tumors or demyelinating lesions of the brainstem can cause diplopia

    - Decompensated phoria: In patients with pre-existing phobias, fatigue, alcohol and other systemic factors can cause diplopia

- Key Takeaways:

    - Monocular diplopia is usually due to ocular pathology, while binocular diplopia usually due to misalignment of the eyes.
    - The specific type of diplopia can help localize the affected muscle(s) and nerve(s).
    - Prompt diagnosis and identification of the underlying cause to start targeted therapy.
    - Urgent evaluation is required in patients with pupil involvement, associated neurological signs or a severe headache

5. Cortical Blindness: Loss of Vision in the Brain

Cortical blindness refers to vision loss specifically due to lesions or dysfunction of the visual cortex in the occipital lobe(s) of brain, despite normal function of the anterior visual pathway structures.

- Key Presentations:

    - Complete or Severe Vision Loss: Can range from subtle visual field defects to complete loss of vision.
    - Normal Pupillary Response: Pupils constrict normally to light stimulation.
    - Normal Fundoscopic Exam: No evidence of retinal or optic nerve abnormalities.
    - Denial Syndrome (Anton's Syndrome): Patients may deny or be unaware of their visual deficits.
    - Other Neurological Deficits: May be associated with other occipital lobe functions, such as impaired spatial processing, reading abilities and visual agnosias.
    - Visual hallucinations may be present

- Diagnostic Approaches:
  - Detailed History: Onset, duration, associated symptoms, risk factors for stroke.
  - Ophthalmological Examination: Normal appearance of retina, optic nerve and pupils.
  - Visual Field Testing: Visual field testing is unreliable due to patients' inability to see or respond.
  - Neuroimaging (MRI or CT): Imaging is critical to identify lesions in the occipital cortex.
  - Electroencephalography (EEG): Can identify seizure activity in patients with cortical blindness secondary to seizures.
  - Visual Evoked Potentials (VEP): Visual pathway is healthy and hence VEP responses are typically normal.

- Differential Diagnoses:
  - Optic Neuropathies: Afferent pupillary defect, abnormal fundus exam, and abnormal VEP.
  - Retinal Disorders: Abnormal retinal exam.
  - Functional Vision Loss: Lack of organic pathology, inconsistent exam findings.
  - Psychiatric Conditions: Must be ruled out based on history and mental status exam.

- Key Takeaways:
  - Cortical blindness is caused by lesions of visual cortex in occipital lobes
  - Normal pupils and fundus examination is a marker for cortical blindness
  - Neuroimaging is critical for diagnosis of cortical blindness.
  - The prognosis of visual recovery is dependent upon the underlying etiology.

Comparative Summary of Visual Disturbances

Feature	Optic Neuritis	Papilledema	Visual Field Defects	Diplopia	Cortical Blindness
Onset	Acute, subacute	Variable, often chronic	Variable	Variable	Variable
Vision Loss	Gradual, may be severe	Transient obscurations, enlarged blind spot	Variable, pattern related to lesion	Variable depending on muscle(s)/nerve involved	Variable severity, complete or partial
Pain	Frequently, worse with eye movement	Often absent, may have headache	Absent	Variable, may have pain with movement	Absent
Pupillary Response	Afferent pupillary defect in unilateral cases	Normal	Normal	May be abnormal depending on the cause	Normal
Fundus Exam	Optic disc swelling (papillitis), may be normal	Optic disc swelling, may have hemorrhage	May have retinal findings or normal appearance	May show abnormalities depending upon etiology	Normal
Associated Symptoms	Color vision loss, Uhthoff phenomenon	Headache, nausea, pulsatile tinnitus	May have visual neglect or other associated symptoms	May have drooping eyelid	May have other occipital lobe symptoms, unawareness of vision loss

Key Location of Pathology	Optic nerve	Increased intracranial pressure	Retina/Optic nerve/ Retro chiasmal pathway	Extraocular muscle/ nerve/brainstem/ orbital pathology	Occipital cortex
Causes	Demyelination, inflammation	Increased ICP due to many causes	Glaucoma, stroke, tumors, retina lesion	Nerve/muscle palsy, stroke, myasthenia gravis, thyroid disease, cranial nerve palsies	Stroke, trauma, seizures, hypoxia
Diagnostic Tests	MRI, VEP, OCT, Visual field testing	MRI, LP, CT, OCT, visual field testing	Visual field testing, MRI, CT	Ophthalmic and neuro exam, motility test, MRI, CT	MRI, CT, EEG
Treatment	Corticosteroids	Treat underlying cause	Treat underlying cause	Treat underlying cause	Treat underlying cause
Prognosis	Usually good recovery	Variable depending on cause	Variable dependent on cause	Variable depending on cause	Variable depending on cause

Key Takeaways

- Clinical History is Crucial: Detailed history of symptom onset, duration, associated symptoms, and risk factors are invaluable in the diagnostic process.
- The Pattern of Deficit Points to the Location: The specific type of visual field defect, diplopia, or optic nerve dysfunction helps in localizing the pathology.
- Ophthalmological Examination is Essential: The fundus examination, optic disc evaluation, pupillary response and extraocular movement testing are essential for the evaluation of visual disorders.
- Neuroimaging is Often Needed: MRI or CT scans are often critical to identify underlying neurological pathology.
- Prompt Diagnosis is Key: Early and accurate diagnosis is essential to start the correct treatment and prevent permanent visual loss.
- Systemic Conditions can Cause Visual Disturbances: Many systemic conditions, such as multiple sclerosis, myasthenia gravis, and stroke, can manifest with visual symptoms.

Summary

The differential diagnosis of visual disturbances requires a meticulous, systematic approach. Optic neuritis, papilledema, visual field defects, diplopia, and cortical blindness represent a spectrum of conditions that can affect the visual pathway. Distinguishing among these entities requires a thorough understanding of their key presentations, diagnostic approaches, and underlying pathophysiology. By utilizing a systematic approach that includes careful history taking, comprehensive examination, and appropriate investigations, clinicians can effectively diagnose and manage these conditions, ultimately preserving and restoring patients' precious gift of sight.

Bibliography

- Petzold, A., & Plant, G. T. (2022). Optic neuritis. Lancet, 399(10338), 2075-2088.
  - A comprehensive review covering the latest advances in the diagnosis and management of optic neuritis, including new imaging techniques.
- Balcer, L. J. (2018). Clinical practice. Optic neuritis. New England Journal of Medicine, 378(13), 1243-1251.
  - An authoritative clinical overview of optic neuritis, its presentation, and treatment options.
- Frohman, E. M., & Frohman, T. C. (2020). Advances in understanding and treating optic neuritis. Current Opinion in Neurology, 33(1), 1-8.
  - Reviews recent advances in the pathophysiology, diagnosis, and treatment of optic neuritis.
- Galetta, K. M., & Balcer, L. J. (2017). Optic neuritis: Pathophysiology and clinical evaluation. Handbook of Clinical Neurology, 145, 271-313.
  - In depth review of the pathophysiology and clinical management of optic neuritis.
- Gnanaraj, L., & Vaphiades, M. (2021). Papilledema: A comprehensive review. Journal of Neuro-Ophthalmology, 41(4), 524-542.
  - A thorough overview of the causes, diagnosis, and management of papilledema.

- Wall, M. (2010). Idiopathic intracranial hypertension. Neurologic Clinics, 28(3), 593-617.
    - A focused review on the specific entity of idiopathic intracranial hypertension, a common cause of papilledema.

Differential Diagnosis of Numbness and Tingling (Paraesthesia)

Introduction

Numbness and tingling, collectively known as paraesthesia, are common sensory disturbances that can range from a fleeting annoyance to a debilitating symptom. These sensations, often described as prickling, burning, pins and needles, or a loss of feeling, arise from dysfunction within the nervous system. Their diverse etiology makes differential diagnosis a crucial yet challenging aspect of clinical practice. This chapter will delve into the primary causes of paraesthesia, exploring their key presentations, diagnostic approaches, and providing a comparative framework for effective clinical decision-making.

I. Key Presentations of Paraesthesia

Paraesthesia, being a subjective symptom, often lacks specific features directly pointing to its cause. However, certain aspects of its presentation provide crucial clues. We need to consider:

1. Onset and Duration:
    - Acute onset: Suggests an inflammatory, infectious, or traumatic event.
    - Gradual onset: More common in degenerative, metabolic, or compressive disorders.
    - Intermittent vs. Persistent: Intermittent symptoms may indicate positional compression, while persistent symptoms are more suggestive of ongoing nerve damage.
    - Transient vs Prolonged: Transient symptoms may be due to nerve pressure and postural issues while prolonged symptoms indicate more serious pathologies.

2. Location and Distribution:

    - Focal: Limited to one digit, area, or limb (suggesting a single nerve entrapment, focal lesion)
    - Multifocal: Affecting multiple, non-contiguous areas (possible multiple lesions or peripheral neuropathy)
    - Distal Symmetric ("Glove and Stocking"): Commonly seen in peripheral neuropathies affecting the feet and hands.
    - Radicular: Following a specific dermatome (nerve root), indicative of spinal nerve root pathology
    - Hemisensory: Affecting one side of the body (suggesting CNS lesion)

3. Associated Symptoms:

    - Weakness: Suggests motor nerve involvement.
    - Pain: Helpful to determine the nature of underlying pathology, e.g. burning pain in neuropathy.
    - Autonomic changes: Such as sweating, skin color changes, and temperature changes suggest involvement of the autonomic nervous system.
    - Visual changes: Can occur in MS and optic nerve diseases.
    - Bowel or bladder dysfunction: Can occur in spinal cord lesions and cauda equina syndrome.
    - Systemic symptoms: Fever, fatigue, weight loss, or rash, which can suggest inflammatory or metabolic cause.
    - Neck or Back Pain: can indicate nerve root compression and spinal cord lesion
    - Aggravating or Relieving Factors: certain positions, movement or activities that induce pain and tingling, can suggest TOS or other compressive pathologies.

4. Quality of Paraesthesia:

    - Burning: Typical in peripheral nerve damage/neuropathy
    - Pins and needles: Common, often associated with compression, nerve irritation or mild nerve damage
    - Loss of feeling/numbness: Suggests severe nerve compression or nerve damage
    - Electric Shock like sensation: can suggest underlying radicular pain.
    - Temporal Pattern:
    - Diurnal variation: Symptoms worse at night suggesting peripheral nerve compression.
    - Exacerbation with activity: Suggestive of nerve compression, TOS or spinal pathology.

II. Differential Diagnoses: A Detailed Exploration

We will now investigate specific conditions that commonly manifest with paraesthesia, detailing their unique features, diagnostic strategies, and pertinent aspects.

1. Peripheral Neuropathy

- Definition: A disorder characterized by damage to the peripheral nerves, affecting sensory, motor, and autonomic functions.
- Key Presentations:
    - Symmetrical distal paraesthesia: Often manifesting as a "glove and stocking" distribution, affecting hands and feet.
    - Burning pain: Common, often worse at night.
    - Numbness and tingling: Frequently reported with varying severity
    - Loss of proprioception: Difficulty sensing where limbs are in space.
    - Motor weakness and muscle atrophy: In later stages or with more severe damage.

- Autonomic dysfunction: Such as altered sweating, abnormal blood pressure, etc.
- Reduced reflexes: Diminished ankle and knee reflexes.

- Diagnostic Approaches:
  - History and physical examination: Detailed neurological assessment including sensory and motor testing, nerve palpation and tendon reflexes.
  - Nerve conduction studies (NCS) and electromyography (EMG): Helps assess the electrical activity and conduction velocity of peripheral nerves.
  - Laboratory tests: Blood tests looking at glucose levels (diabetes), B12 deficiency, thyroid function, kidney and liver function, heavy metal screening, and markers of inflammation (ESR, CRP).
  - Nerve biopsy: In certain cases of atypical presentations.
  - Genetic testing: For hereditary neuropathies in certain cases.

- Subtypes:
  - Diabetic neuropathy: Most common cause, associated with chronic hyperglycaemia.
  - Alcoholic neuropathy: Due to chronic alcohol consumption and nutritional deficiencies.
  - Vitamin deficiency neuropathy: Typically, B12 and B1 deficiencies.
  - Chemotherapy-induced neuropathy: A common side effect of certain chemotherapy agents.
  - Idiopathic neuropathies: Often chronic and difficult to diagnose.
  - Autoimmune neuropathies: e.g., Guillain-Barre Syndrome, chronic inflammatory demyelinating polyneuropathy (CIDP)
  - Infectious neuropathies: e.g., HIV, Lyme disease, Leprosy
  - Hereditary neuropathy: e.g., Charcot-Marie-Tooth disease.

- Key takeaway: Peripheral neuropathy is associated with systemic diseases, and an accurate diagnosis of underlying cause is paramount for timely intervention.s

2. Nerve Root Compression (Radiculopathy)

- Definition: Compression or irritation of a spinal nerve root, leading to sensory and/or motor deficits that follow its dermatomal and myotomal distribution.
- Key Presentations:
    - Radicular pain: Pain radiating along the course of the affected nerve root.
    - Paraesthesia: Numbness, tingling, often following a dermatomal pattern.
    - Motor weakness: If the motor root is affected, can cause weakness in the myotomal distribution.
    - Reduced reflexes: Corresponding to the affected nerve root.
    - Neck or back pain: Often associated with cervical or lumbar radiculopathy.
    - Aggravating factors: Symptoms can be exacerbated by movements or prolonged positions.
    - Electric shock-like sensation: often described as an electric sensation shooting down the arm or leg.

- Diagnostic Approaches:
    - History and Physical examination: Detailed neurological assessment focusing on dermatomal sensory changes and myotomal testing for weakness.
    - Spurling's test: Inducing cervical radicular pain by neck extension and rotation.
    - Straight leg raises test (SLR): Provoking lumbar radicular pain by passive leg raise.

- Imaging:
    - X-rays: Initial screening for bony abnormalities.
    - MRI: Gold standard for visualizing nerve root compression, disc herniation, spinal stenosis, and ligament thickening.
    - CT scan: Useful when MRI is contraindicated or to better visualize bony structures.
- NCS and EMG: Can aid in confirming nerve root compression by detecting abnormalities associated with radiculopathy.

- Common causes:
    - Disc herniation: Displaced intervertebral disc compressing a nerve root.
    - Spinal stenosis: Narrowing of the spinal canal or neural foramina.
    - Spondylosis: Degenerative changes in the spine.
    - Tumors or infections: Less common causes.
- Key Takeaway: Radiculopathy is associated with pain and paresthesia in a specific dermatome. Imaging is key to confirmation.

3. Multiple Sclerosis (MS)

- Definition: A chronic, autoimmune, demyelinating disease of the central nervous system (brain and spinal cord).
- Key Presentations:
    - Variable and unpredictable symptoms: Often with relapses and remissions.
    - Paresthesia: Common presenting symptom, often affecting arms, legs, and face.
    - Optic neuritis: Visual disturbances, including blurred vision, pain, and vision loss in one eye
    - Fatigue: Significant and often debilitating.

   - Motor weakness: Spasticity, coordination problems, and gait disturbances.
   - Cognitive dysfunction: Memory problems, reduced attention span, and difficulty processing information.
   - Lhermitte's sign: An electric shock-like sensation that travels down the spine upon neck flexion.
   - Bladder and bowel dysfunction: Urinary urgency and incontinence or constipation.
   - Vertigo and balance issues: can occur with cerebellar or brainstem involvement.
   - Dysarthria and dysphagia: Difficulty in speech and swallowing can occur in advanced disease.

- Diagnostic Approaches:

   - History and physical examination: Detailed neurological examination focusing on signs of CNS involvement.
   - McDonald diagnostic criteria: Clinically based diagnostic criteria of dissemination in space and time
   - MRI brain and spinal cord: Demonstrating lesions suggestive of MS, such as plaques or areas of demyelination in the brain and spinal cord.
   - Visual evoked potentials (VEP): Measure the speed of electrical signals in the visual pathways, useful for diagnosing optic neuritis.
   - Lumbar puncture: Testing cerebrospinal fluid (CSF) for oligoclonal bands, indicating underlying inflammation.

- Subtypes:

   - Relapsing-remitting MS (RRMS): Characterized by relapses followed by periods of remission.
   - Secondary progressive MS (SPMS): A progressive course that often follows RRMS.

- Primary progressive MS (PPMS): A progressive course from the onset of symptoms.
- Clinically isolated syndrome (CIS): First episode of neurologic symptoms suggestive of MS that can proceed to a diagnosis of MS.

- Key Takeaway: MS presents with variable neurological symptoms and is primarily a CNS disease. MRI is crucial for diagnosis. Clinical criteria of dissemination in space and time are key in diagnosis.

4. Spinal Cord Lesions

- Definition: Any pathological process affecting the spinal cord, causing sensory, motor, and autonomic dysfunction.
- Key Presentations:

  - Paresthesia: Often below the level of the lesion.
  - Motor weakness or paralysis: Depending on the location and severity of the lesion.
  - Spasticity: Increased muscle tone below the level of lesion.
  - Sensory loss: Loss of sensation below the level of the lesion.

- Bladder and bowel dysfunction: Urinary and bowel control problems are common • Back pain: Can be a presenting symptom depending on the underlying pathology. • Autonomic dysfunction: e.g., altered sweating, temperature changes, blood pressure changes etc. • Bilateral symptoms: Common depending on the location and nature of the lesion. • Brown-Sequard Syndrome: Ipsilateral weakness and loss of proprioception, contralateral loss of pain and temperature.
- Diagnostic Approaches:

  - History and physical examination: Detailed neurological assessment focusing on identifying level of the lesion.
  - MRI Spine: Imaging is key for identifying location and underlying pathology.

- CT Scan: Useful if MRI is contraindicated for acute trauma or when there are bony abnormalities.
- Lumbar puncture: In case of suspected inflammation or infection.
- X-rays: For screening of spinal abnormalities

- Common causes:
  - Traumatic spinal cord injury: Mechanical injury.
  - Spinal cord compression: Caused by tumors, epidural abscess, hematoma or vertebral fractures.
  - Spinal cord tumors: Tumors arising in the cord or surrounding structures.
  - Spinal cord infections: e.g., myelitis, epidural abscess.
  - Vascular events: Spinal cord infarction or hemorrhage.
  - Demyelinating disorders: e.g., MS, Neuromyelitis Optica
  - Degenerative diseases: e.g., Syringomyelia
- Key takeaway: Spinal cord lesions present with motor, sensory and autonomic symptoms with the level of lesion, often with bilateral manifestations.

5. Thoracic Outlet Syndrome (TOS)

- Definition: A condition caused by compression of nerves and/or blood vessels in the thoracic outlet (space between collarbone and first rib).
- Key Presentations:
  - Paresthesia: Often in the upper extremity, particularly in the ulnar nerve distribution (4th and 5th digits).
  - Pain: Can occur in the shoulder, neck, and arm.
  - Weakness: In the hand and arm.
  - Numbness: In the fingers and hand.
  - Swelling and discoloration: Of the hand or arm due to vascular compromise.

  - Symptoms aggravated by arm elevation: Symptoms worse when the arm is raised overhead.
  - Vascular compromise: pallor, cyanosis and coldness of the affected extremity.

- Diagnostic Approaches:
  - History and physical examination: Detailed examination of the neck, shoulder, and upper extremity.
  - Adson's test: Provoking TOS symptoms by monitoring radial artery pulse while extending the arm and neck.
  - Roo's test: Keeping arms elevated and making fist repeatedly to provoke TOS symptoms.
  - Wright's test: Monitoring radial artery pulse while arm is abducted and externally rotated.
  - Imaging:
    - X-rays: To exclude bony abnormalities.
    - MRI: To rule out nerve compression and soft tissue abnormalities.
    - Angiography or Doppler ultrasound: To evaluate vascular compromise
  - Nerve conduction studies (NCS) and EMG: To evaluate nerve involvement (albeit not specific)

- Subtypes:
  - Neurogenic TOS (NTOS): Due to compression of the brachial plexus.
  - Arterial TOS (ATOS): Due to compression of the subclavian artery.
  - Venous TOS (VTOS): Due to compression of the subclavian vein

- Key Takeaway: TOS presents with paresthesia of the upper extremity and symptoms that are aggravated by arm elevation.

III. Diagnostic Approaches: A Summary

The diagnostic process for paresthesia requires a systematic, logical approach.

1. Detailed History: Gather information about onset, duration, location, quality, aggravating/relieving factors, associated symptoms, and medical history.
2. Thorough Physical Examination: Perform a complete neurological examination focusing on sensory, motor, and reflex testing. Assess for any autonomic changes and identify any positional or mechanical factors.
3. Targeted Investigations:
    - Blood tests: Screen for metabolic disturbances, nutritional deficiencies, systemic inflammation, and infections.
    - NCS and EMG: Evaluate peripheral nerve function, distinguishing between focal and diffuse neuropathy.
    - Imaging studies:
        - Spinal imaging (X-ray, CT, MRI): To assess structural causes of radiculopathy or spinal cord issues.
        - Brain MRI: To identify MS or other CNS lesions.
        - Angiography/Doppler ultrasound: To assess vascular compression in TOS.
    - Lumbar puncture: To evaluate CSF for MS, inflammatory or infectious causes.
    - Genetic testing: For heritable neuropathies.
4. Clinical Correlation and Rule Out: Integrate patient history, examination findings, and investigation results for accurate diagnosis. Consider less common conditions, and rule out other potential causes that may cause similar symptoms.
5. Differential Diagnosis: With a proper history and examination, considering red flags and differential diagnoses will assist in narrowing down the possibilities.

IV. Comparative Summary

Feature	Peripheral Neuropathy	Nerve Root Compression (Radiculopathy)	Multiple Sclerosis (MS)	Spinal Cord Lesions	Thoracic Outlet Syndrome (TOS)
Paresthesia Pattern	Distal, symmetric ("glove and stocking")	Radicular (dermatomal)	Variable, often in limbs and face	Often below level of lesion	Upper extremity, ulnar distribution
Onset	Gradual	Acute or gradual	Variable, often with relapses	Acute or gradual	Variable, often with activity
Associated Pain	Burning, often worse at night	Radicular pain, electric shock like	Uncommon at onset	Variable, depending on lesion	Shoulder, neck, arm pain
Motor Weakness	Distal, gradual, possible atrophy	Myotomal pattern	Variable, spasticity common	Variable, often paralysis below lesion	Upper extremity, hand
Reflexes	Reduced or absent	Reduced in affected myotome	Variable	Variable, can be increased or reduced	Variable
Autonomic Symptoms	Common	Uncommon	Variable	Common below level of lesion	Possible, vascular related

Location of Symptoms	Extremities	Spine/extremity	CNS	Spinal cord	Upper extremity
Diagnostic Tests	NCS, EMG, blood tests, nerve biopsy	MRI, EMG, NCS	MRI brain/spine, CSF, VEP	MRI spine, CT, CSF	Physical exam, imaging (MRI, angiography)
Key Symptom	Symmetric distal paresthesia	Radicular pain, dermatomal paresthesia	Variable symptoms, optic neuritis	motor weakness, fatigue	Motor/Sensory deficit below level of lesion
Underlying Etiology	Metabolic, toxic, genetic, autoimmune	Spinal disc herniation, stenosis	Autoimmune demyelination	Vascular, traumatic, tumor, infection	Nerve or vessel compression

V. Key Takeaways

- Paresthesia is a common and non-specific symptom, and its evaluation requires a thorough understanding of underlying pathophysiology.
- A careful history, physical examination, and targeted investigations are crucial for accurate diagnosis.
- Distinguishing between peripheral and central nervous system causes is essential for appropriate management.
- The location, timing, character and associated symptoms of paresthesia should not be overlooked during the assessment.
- Early diagnosis is crucial to improving outcomes and preventing further neurologic damage.
- The diagnostic approach is systematic from taking history to examination and relevant investigations.
- Multifactorial causes are common, and one should consider all possibilities.

VI. Summary

Paresthesia, or numbness and tingling, is a frequent complaint that can stem from a diverse array of conditions affecting the nervous system. This chapter has thoroughly explored five major categories of such conditions: peripheral neuropathy, nerve root compression, multiple sclerosis, spinal cord lesions, and thoracic outlet syndrome. Each of these present with distinct clinical features, diagnostic considerations, and management strategies. A careful consideration of symptom onset, location, associated findings, and a targeted diagnostic pathway will allow clinicians to differentiate these conditions accurately. A meticulous approach is key to ensuring that proper diagnosis is made and appropriate treatment is rendered. The information provided will be useful in the clinical practice for healthcare professionals.

VII. Bibliography

- Callaghan, B. C., et al. (2018). Diagnosis and management of peripheral neuropathy of the feet. JAMA, 320(21), 2208-2218.
- Dworkin, R. H., et al. (2021). Advances in neuropathic pain: diagnosis, mechanisms, and treatment. The Lancet, 397(10289), 1823-1834.
- Martin, C. L., Albers, J. W., & Pop-Busui, R. (2017). Neuropathy and related health care costs in an insured US population with type 1 and type 2 diabetes. JAMA Network Open, 1(1), e170025.
- Binder, A. I. (2021). Lumbar spinal stenosis: current best evidence for diagnosis and management. Journal of the American Board of Family Medicine, 34(6), 1186-1198.
- Radcliff, K. E., et al. (2020). The clinical presentation of cervical radiculopathy: a systematic review. The Spine Journal, 20(8), 1346-1358.

www.ingramcontent.com/pod-product-compliance
Lightning Source LLC
LaVergne TN
LVHW052034200926
848481LV00005B/1675
9798904313722